a

b

The Value of Agroforestry for Livestock in the Tropics

Luis Orlando Alba Gomez, PhD

Full Professor and Consulting Professor
Discipline: Reproduction and Genetics

Notice

This is a complementary book intended to advise and guide those involved in the development of agroforestry for livestock farming in the tropics. Results may vary for various reasons beyond our control. Therefore, we cannot be held responsible for actions carried out on farms without our supervision.

The Value of Agroforestry for Livestock in the Tropics

Copyright 2024 by Luis Orlando Alba Gomez
Cover Designer: Igor Alba Espinosa
Style review: Igor Alba Espinosa

All rights reserved

No part of this publication may be reproduced or transmitted in any form or by any means, electronic or mechanical, without the written permission of the publisher.

Printer in the United States of America
Edited by Amazon Kindle Direct Publishing

Dedication

To my children and to all those who collaborated in one way or another in the completion of this work

Acknowledgements

I particularly deserve my thanks to the many graduate students whom I guided scientifically in serious scientific-student activities, such as Coursework, Diploma Theses or in postgraduate activities such as Specialization and Doctoral Theses. The list of graduates would be too long to reproduce here, but many of their names appear in the references at the end of this book.

Preface

This book has been designed to present an updated and suitable summary of the bibliography regarding the agroecological and zootechnical actions that have been affecting tropical livestock and whose results remain dispersed in libraries, which are difficult to access for most interested readers. It also serves the purpose of providing technicians, livestock breeders and professionals in the field with a useful source of information on the altering effects of the tropical climate on animal economy and the ways to improve livestock ecosystems through agrosilvipastoral cultivation methods.

Its main virtues are the agroecological and zootechnical approaches that are offered to solve the problems of self-sufficiency of food for animals, together with the regulation of the agroecological and zootechnical actions that are presented to improve the reproductive and productive efficiency of cattle.

Content

Preface		g
Introduction		1
Cap.1	**The livestock agro-ecosystem in the tropics**	3
	Results and deficiencies in commertial production	4
	Agroecosystems and regionalization of plants	6
	Alternatives of pastures and forages for tropics farms	8
	Conservation of pastures and forages	34
	Limitations of the use of standars in dairy cattle	43
	Contribution of agroforestry to food self sufficiency	46
	Results of the introduction of the silvi-pastoral system in live farms	58
Cap.2	**Effects of the tropical climate on animal economy**	63
	Tropical climate as a limiting factor	64
	General characterists of the tropical climate	67
	Environmental stress in animals	80
	Soil and its conservation	88
Cap.3	**Adjustment and evaluation of zootechnical actions**	90
	Selection of heifers for replacement	91
	Reproductive management in breeding livestock	95
	Evaluation of reproductive performance of herd	108
	Interpretation of reproductive indices	112
Cap.4	**Proposal for an agroforestry project**	124
Bibliography		142
Author's review		146

Introduction

The limiting factors that most affect the development of livestock farming in the tropics are the poor soils and the dry period that means months of scarcity for animal feed.

The study of the annual distribution of the energy provided by pasture shows the critical food situation that occurs in the months of December to April, and sometimes May, even with cultivated pastures.

Therefore, livestock systems, totally dependent on the spontaneous production of pasture, have low productivity rates. These systems, linked to nature and regional traditions, are very inefficient from the productive point of view.

In this sense, what was expressed by the French zootechnician André-M. Leroy, in his book Rational Livestock Breeding (1967), when he compared the breeding methods used in underdeveloped countries in the African tropics with those in Europe, is still valid.

"If we now consider what happens on an important farm in Normandy or Flanders, we will be surprised by the complexity of the care applied to livestock. We will see, first, that the animals are housed during bad weather in spacious stables which protect them from rain and cold. The haylofts are filled with good hay, intended for winter feeding.

This reserve of fodder is completed by beets or other roots, specially cultivated for use in the bad season. From birth, the calves are fed a carefully prepared diet, according to their age, weight and appetite. Milk is not skimped on, at least during the first few weeks."

This comparison could be extended to the livestock of many countries in the world a century later. So, if the solution is to prepare for the bad season, why not do so using existing local natural resources?

Chapter 1

The livestock agro-ecosystem in the tropics

Contents:
Introduction. Results and deficiencies in commercial production. Agro-ecosystems and regionalization of plants. Alternative of pastures and forages existing in the tropics for the food self-sufficiency of farms. Conservation of pastures and forages. Limitations of the use of standards in dairy cattle. Contribution of agroforestry to food self-sufficiency. Regionalization of trees to improve ecosystems. Results of the introduction of the silvi-pastoral system in livestock farms. Conditions for planting trees in livestock systems.

Introduction

The food base of cattle farming in the tropics must be based on the intensive use of pastures and forages and, therefore, the reconversion of the production system must be oriented towards the benefit of a food base of its own with food resources generated on the farm, based on the soil and climate conditions, the genotype of the cattle and the use of the available natural resources. It is necessary to define the most suitable areas for each component, considering the factors that are considered most significant for the success of the company.

Results and deficiencies in commercial production

It is generally agreed that the food base of cattle farming in the tropics must be based on the intensive use of pastures and forages and, therefore, the conversion of the production system must be oriented towards the development of a food base of its own, with the food resources generated on the farm, based on the soil and climate conditions, genotype of the cattle and use of human, material and natural resources. However, the goal of achieving a balanced diet throughout the year has encountered numerous difficulties.

Traditionally, tropical cattle farming has been governed by a kind of climatic fatalism, in which the least rainy period of the year is equivalent to an increase in empty cows, functional anestrus, a drastic decrease in milk production and chronic malnutrition, which causes delayed puberty in heifers, predisposition to diseases and in extreme cases death, in all categories of cattle.

The general trend has been to obtain meat and milk from cattle, without investing enough in food production and other important inputs for their well-being and survival in periods of scarcity.

There has been no due agro-technical attention to natural or cultivated pastures (fertilizers, irrigation) or other actions to improve the conditions of the livestock agroecosystem.

Subjective factors include the attitude of many cattle farmers of not wanting to produce food for their animals, ignorance of the advantages of new technologies for planting and preserving food, and also the refusal to accept an additional, more arduous and less remunerative work process.

For the reasons mentioned above, agricultural professionals and technicians must play a leading role in achieving the commitment, understanding and acceptance by cattle farmers of a complex production system based on biological processes, where extension, training and remuneration for farm profits are essential elements.

The creation of a food base of its own, where sugar cane, cultivated pastures, protein banks, fodder trees, hay and silage play essential roles, constitutes the most important challenge to achieve technological reconversion and real food self-sufficiency.

Agroecosystems and regionalization of plants

The study of species adaptation to particular ecosystems is currently referred to as livestock agroecosystems and can be considered the wisest way to approach nature's models.

To define livestock agroecosystems, aspects such as climate behavior, animal species, breeds, productive purpose, herd size, exploitation technologies, existing pastures, soil types, limiting factors, agro-productive categories and some agro-socioeconomic considerations are considered, including aspects of the livestock culture of the environment and the existing infrastructure to carry out production.

Regionalizing

Is selecting the species or varieties that are suitable for each place where they are going to be sown.

Place

Understanding by place not only the physical area of the land, but something much broader known as an **ecosystem**, which is the result of a balanced combination of all the factors that intervene in the **soil-plant-animal-man** complex in which all the aspects that affect the production, use and permanence of the grass have an impact and are related, differentiating itself from other ecosystems either by the soil or the climate where they are exploited; or by the inputs that are destined for the soil or the animal; or by the purpose that is pursued and also by the way in which man manages them.

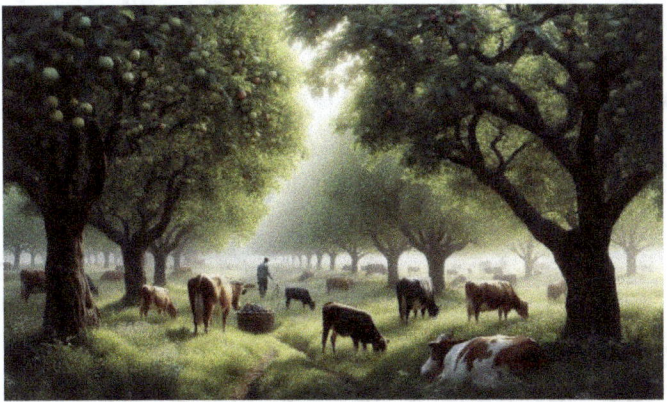

Figure 1 shows the relationship and the factors involved in the soil-plant-animal-man complex.

Alternatives of pastures and forages existing in the tropics for the food self-sufficiency of farms

Currently, a total of 27 species and accessions of grasses and 16 of legumes are regionalized according to soil conditions, rainfall and management (load, fertilization and purpose). Of all of them, reference will be made to the most useful ones.

Below, I will present a list of grasses and legumes and their main virtues and defects, which aims to demonstrate the numerous alternatives that exist to achieve food self-sufficiency in state and private farms, and to improve the livestock agro-system, according to the characteristics of the region in question.

Most of the data was taken from the Manual of Technologies for the Promotion and Exploitation of Pastures and Forages, by Gabriel Oquendo Lobaina and from works from the Experimental Stations of Pastures and Forages of Havana, Indio Hatuey de Matanzas, Sancti Spiritus and Holguín, with the advantage that the cultivation technologies and their results were obtained under production conditions and using participatory methods, to avoid gross mistakes when extending them on a large scale.

Grasses

A. gayanus cv CIAT-621 (Gamba grass)

This grass has a very high natural reseeding power and a great capacity to produce seeds. It has a vigorous and deep root system and its resistance to drought allows it to persist for a long time.

Due to its high dry matter content, when used as cut fodder it can produce 12 to 20 tons per hectare per year. When grazed, it can withstand loads of up to 2,5-4.0 adult cattle per hectare even in low fertilization and no irrigation conditions.

It has a good taste, but its nutritional value is relatively low, from medium to low, so it is recommended to sow it in association with leguminous plants. It is best used to feed developing animals, beef biotype cattle or cows with medium dairy potential.

A. gayanus is an ideal species to sow in poor soils, lacking phosphorus and abundant in aluminum. Under these conditions it can perform better than *Panicum*, *Brachiaria* and *Cynodon* species. It is not demanding in terms of irrigation or fertilizers, although it responds well to applications in medium doses.

Dactylon. (Bermuda grass)

It adapts to a wide variety of soils, including saline and poorly drained soils.

All these varieties of grass can be used to make excellent hay and are suitable for ensiling. In addition, they are very desirable for livestock both as forage and direct grazing.

Brachiaria spp

In Cuba, *B. purpuracens* cv Aguada (formerly *Brizantha*) is currently planted and *Brachiaria mutica* (para grass) grows spontaneously. *B. decumbens* CIAT-606, *B. humidicola* CIAT-679; *Brachiaria Brizantha* (marandu=brizanton=*brachiaron*) and *B. dyctioneura* are promising.

These species are not demanding in terms of irrigation and only require medium or low levels of fertilizer, depending on the degree of consumption to which they are to be subjected. All varieties can be used as cut or grazed forage, but *B. purpuracens* is better as cut forage and *B. humidicola* for grazing by growing animals. It is recommended to associate these species with similar leguminous plants, particularly kudzu, arachis and others.

Cenchrus ciliaris cvs Biloela. (Buffel, Formidable)

These species adapt well to soils of various textures, except those with high clay; they prefer light soils, rich in calcium, with neutral or alkaline pH, but they resist poor drainage or prolonged waterlogging. They do not have high fertilization requirements, nor do they need irrigation, although they respond well to both practices.

These cultivars have a good yield and quality potential, so they can be used both for cutting for hay and for grazing for growing animals and for cows with medium dairy potential.

Saccharum officinarum L. (Sugar cane)

Contrary to what one might think, sugar cane is the main forage species used at a national level and is the best forage in terms of the benefits it offers to the current livestock ecosystem: the yields per unit area are greater than any other tropical forage, it does not lose quality with age, it is harvested in the least rainy period, cutting, transporting and other agricultural tasks are done manually and with animal traction; in suitable soils it is not demanding in terms of irrigation, it responds well to organic fertilization and cultural work and in general its exploitation technology is traditional knowledge for the producer.

It can be used as compensation forage, chopped together with the green leaves; The bud and green leaves are used to make good silage, and the ground stem can be used to obtain rustic saccharina. All of this is done in the production unit itself.

Forage varieties

The National Institute of Sugarcane Technologies of Cuba recommends propagating the following 21 genotypes in the different livestock areas: B80250, C128-83, C132-81, C137-81, C85-203, C86-12, C86-165, C86-503, C86-536, C87-252, C87-51, C88-553, C89-161, C89-176, C90-317, C90-501, C90-530, C91-356, C92-203, C95-416, Co997.

These varieties are characterized by their resistance to diseases typical of this species and by having a high forage value, with more than 50 % dry matter digestibility.

The varieties C86-505, C90-530, C90-317, C89-176, C86-165 and C86-12 are suitable for use in poor soils and in areas with low rainfall.

The varieties C86-12, C86-503, Co997, C137-81 and C132-81 are more suitable for use in poorly drained soils.

The varieties not recommended due to their low digestibility are: Ja 60-5 40,0; PR 980 33,5; My 5718 30,1; C 1984-74 27,0; C 751-75 26,4.

P. maximun cvs likoni, and *Uganda.* (Guinea)

These grasses are very leafy, grow in clumps and have an erect habit. They have a wide and deep root system, which makes them resistant to drought. They also tolerate the shade of trees, shrubs and companion plants.

Compared to other species, they have a high DM yield, are very palatable and have a high nutritional value. They can withstand cutting every 6-12 weeks to produce forage or silage but are better for direct grazing with any animal category.

Common guinea grass has been naturalized in Cuba since the 16th century and is adapted to all regions of the country. Currently, the likoni variety is also used, which has the property of establishing itself more quickly, being more efficient in natural rehabilitation and producing more and better seeds than *P. maximun* itself.

There are other commercial cultivars, SIH-127 obtained at the Indio Hatuey Pasture and Forage Station and the so-called Australian and Uganda varieties. All have good plasticity, high yields and good quality.

Digitaria decumbens. (Pangola grass)

This species has a high nutritional value and can be used for cutting, hay, silage or fresh fodder and for grazing for any category and potential animal.

Although it is very resistant to drought, it does not grow during that time. Its growth can be affected when there is high humidity for prolonged periods.

This species of grass has the difficulty of being susceptible to the attack of rust (*Puccinia sp*), which can completely damage it.

Cynodon nlemfuensis. (Star grass)

This grass is very invasive, with creeping growth, with thick and very vigorous stolons up to 4 m long. It adapts to almost all types of soils with different pH.

It can be used both for cutting and for grazing; but it is not good for haymaking.

It is not very demanding in terms of irrigation and fertilization, although it responds well to its application. Its efficiency in nutrient assimilation, together with its rusticity, allows it to withstand a greater load than other grasses.

Chloris gayana cv Callide. (Rhodes grass)

It establishes well in various types of soils, except in very acidic and poorly drained soils. It adapts to a pH range of 6.0 to 8.5 and is resistant to salinity.

The Callide variety grows erect, but produces stolon's, which are used to reproduce it vegetatively. It has the property of establishing itself quickly and spreading naturally. It is suitable for producing hay.

Pennisetum purpureum cvs king grass; CRAAG-265; Taiwan 144

Elephant or Napier grass (*Pennisetum purpureum*) in all its varieties, is the most popular species as cutting grass in Cuba. It is easy to establish, grows in any type of soil, responds remarkably quickly to fertilization and when well cared for, lasts indefinitely.

These three cultivars complement King grass (*Saccharum sinese*), but never surpass it in DM yield.

They are generally used for direct fodder or to make silage. They have the quality of containing high levels of soluble carbohydrates, but their DM percentage is low.

Therefore, when used for silage, the addition of cane molasses is not necessary. They can be used for grazing, combined with other species.

Their optimal cutting frequency is 60 days in the rainy season and 90 days in the less rainy season.

These varieties are highly attacked by the false looper pest (*Mocis spp*), which markedly reduces their yield and leaf production.

Cuba CT-115

CT-115 is a fodder plant obtained from King grass in the laboratories of the Cuban Institute of Animal Science, among whose characteristics the following stand out:

a) Greater number of tillers per seedling

b) Higher sugar content

c) Low height due to reduced internode size

d) Better leaf: stem ratio when nodes are shortened

e) It flowers very little

f) It responds well after grazing

Its low flowering period allows it to be left in the field as a food reserve from late spring until the beginning of the dry season, without affecting its quality, which, added to its good proportion of leaves and regrowth capacity, give it (unlike the King grass from which it originated) favorable characteristics for grazing. In two cuts per year (every six months), the total forage it produces can be over 200 t/ha/year.

Zea mays L. (Corn)

Corn is the most widely used grass in developed countries to produce fodder and silage, due to its excellent qualities as a bulky feed. Despite its qualities as a fodder plant, its use in many tropical countries has been extremely limited, due to the deep-rooted tendency of cattle farmers not to plant feed for their cows and because its cultivation is more demanding than other grasses.

From an agro-technical point of view, corn is a plant that requires light, slightly moist and friable soils, although it can be planted in any type of soil with good surface and internal drainage. It does not resist waterlogged soils or soils that are very acidic or alkaline.

The root system of corn is shallow and therefore not very resistant to drought. It has the advantage that it can be planted throughout the year, if irrigation is available.

This grass, because it consumes a lot of soil nutrients, should be fertilized with high levels of N, P and K, preferably at the time of sowing, and its crop should be rotated with leguminous plants.

Corn can yield 90-100 t/ha of green fodder. In sandy and fertilized soils, yields of 60-80 t/ha can be obtained. There are numerous hybrids (HDT–66, HDT–77 and HDT–90) and the varieties Francisco, Rosita, VM–Tuson, vs T-5 and T-6. With them, yields of 3 to 4 t of grain/ha can be obtained.

Sorghum bicolor L. Moench. (Sorghum)

This plant has slightly grooved and oval stems similar to corn. In comparison with the latter, sorghum has less leaf area, but it has a more branched and deeper root system, which gives it greater resistance to drought.

Sorghum grows well in any type of soil with good surface and internal drainage. With good growing conditions, annual yields of 10 to 15 t/ha of DM and 800 to 850 kg/ha of forage can be obtained. For grain sorghum, yields of between 2,5 and 3,0 t/ha can be obtained.

Helianthus annuus. (Sunflower)

The sunflower is an herbaceous plant from the Asteraceae family. It is a crop that is not very demanding in terms of soil type, although it grows better in sandy clay soils rich in organic matter, but the soil must have good drainage and a shallow water table.

The sunflower contains up to 58 % oil in its fruit. This oil is edible and can also be used as fuel (biodiesel). The product remaining after the oil extraction is processed into flour for animal feed.

Legumes

Centrosema pubescens. (Centro or Butterfly pea)

It is a perennial, very vigorous and leafy plant, creeping and climbing, which forms a very dense turf plot.

It grows well in a wide variety of soils, from sandy loam to clayey. But it grows better in reddish brown fersialitic soils.

When irrigated, its DM yield can reach 10-13 t/ha.

When grazed, it can produce 4,0-6,0 t/rotation in the rainy season and 1,2-1,8 t in the dry season. It has given good results when used as a protein bank for developing cattle.

Associated with *Andropogon gayanus*, it constitutes a quality diet for milk production.

Clitoria ternatea. (Blue pea or Bluebellvine)

It is a perennial shrub plant with vigorous growth at its base, but a potential climber if it finds support. It has a dry matter production potential of 10-16 t/ha/year of DM.

Due to its acceptable flavor, it can be used in rotational grazing, associated with grasses such as Napier elephant grass, sorghum and guinea grass. This species has the difficulty of being greatly affected by *Rhizoctonia* and *Cercospora* attacks in high humidity conditions.

Neonotonia wightii. (Glycine or Cooper glycine)

This legume is more demanding with respect to soil quality. These must be fertile, with good drainage and a pH between 6.5-7.0. It does not resist very dry, waterlogged or very acidic soils.

It can be used as forage cut at a height greater than 10 cm with a frequency of 4 to 5 cuts/year and obtain a yield of 12-18 t/ha of DM; however, it is more appropriate for grazing.

It can also be used as a protein bank for dairy cows or associated with grasses for other categories of animals.

Leucaena leucocephala. (Leucaena)

It is a tall shrub that can reach three meters and produces very abundant branches. It has a deep and strong root system that allows it to grow quickly and be resistant to drought.

In pure cultivation it can be used as a protein bank or to produce fodder. As a protein bank it can occupy between 20-30 % of the area and be grazed every 21 to 35 days, for 2 to 3 hours a day during the rainy season and on alternate days with the same schedule during the dry season.

If Leucaena is used as fodder, it can withstand 4-6 cuts at a height of 10-15 cm and produce 12 to 18 t/ha/year of DM with a protein content of 14-20 %.

Moringa oleifera Lam. (Moringa)

Moringa or malungay is a multipurpose tropical tree, native to northern India. It grows in all types of soil, even in drought conditions.

It is a very rustic plant, easy to grow, which stands out for its rapid growth (about three meters in its first year and up to five meters in height in ideal conditions); in its adult state it can reach a maximum height of 10 or 12 m. It flowers 7 months after planting. Its wood is used as firewood and to make charcoal or to convert it into good quality cellulose.

Moringa as fodder is highly nutritious and stands out for a long list of beneficial characteristics, as it is used for cattle, pigs, sheep, goats and poultry, which generates significant increases in both live weight and milk production.

Moringa oleifera, also known as the "*tree of life*" or "*miracle tree*", has been used for centuries for its many medicinal properties and health benefits. Its leaves and seeds are rich in nutrients and are believed to have anti-inflammatory and antioxidant properties. An oil that protects the skin and hair is extracted from its seeds.

It is also used to treat some digestive and liver conditions, and as an antimicrobial.

The taste of Moringa is pleasant and its leaves and flowers can be eaten by humans, raw or cooked and added to stews.

It is one of the plant species with the highest oil content (35%), which makes it an important resource for producing quality biodiesel.

The crop has a yield of 2,500 kg/hectare, which can produce approximately 1,500 liters of oil or more than 1,400 liters of biodiesel/ha.

Azadirachta indica. (Neem, Lilac)

This plant is not a legume or fodder, but is included here for its value as a shade tree and for its medicinal properties.

It is a tree native to India, belonging to the *Meliaceae* family. It grows rapidly and can reach 15 to 20 meters in height.

It develops a lot of foliage in all seasons of the year, but under severe conditions it loses its leaves, even almost completely. The branches are wide and can reach 15 to 20 m in diameter in the fully grown tree.

The leaf stem measures 20 to 40 cm in length, with 20 to 31 dark green leaves 3 to 8 cm long. The flowers, white and fragrant, measure more than 25 cm in length. Its fruit is an olive-like drupe, ranging in shape from an elongated oval to a slightly rounded one, and when ripe it measures 14 mm to 28 mm in length and 10 to 15 mm in width.

The neem tree has a remarkable resistance to drought. It normally survives in areas with semi-arid conditions with a rainfall between 400 mm and 1200 mm. It can develop in regions with a rainfall of less than 400 mm, but in both cases its development depends on the amount of water in the subsoil.

Neem can develop in different types of soil, but it grows best in well-drained, deep and sandy substrates (with a pH of 6.2 to 7). As a species native to tropical and subtropical areas, the tree demands a lot of light and temperatures between 26 °C and 36 °C, preferring deep soils and loam or sandy soils, also accepting a certain degree of salinity.

Due to its medicinal properties, almost all parts of the tree are used as traditional medicine in many countries. The stem, root, and fruits are used as tonics and astringents.

Anti-inflammatory and antibacterial properties:

    a) Neem is used to treat various infections and reduce inflammation.

    b) Diabetes control: It can help reduce blood sugar levels.

c) Strengthening the immune system: It contains compounds that increase the body's ability to fight viruses and bacteria.

d) Skin care: It is effective in treating skin problems such as acne, psoriasis, and eczema.

e) Insect repellent: Neem oil is an active ingredient in many organic insecticidal and fungicidal products.

Stylosanthes guianensis. (Stylo)

It is a perennial herbaceous plant with a taproot that can reach a depth of one meter.

It is a short-day photoperiodic plant and therefore flowers abundantly in the months of December-January. It is very tolerant of low-fertility, acidic or slightly acidic soils.

This legume is ideal for use in association with grasses and is capable of supporting loads of two to four animals/ha, in dry conditions, and obtaining live weight gains of up to 450 kg/ha.

Teramnus labialis. (Teramnus)

It is a perennial plant with a thin stem that has stolon's and basal buds at ground level that are mixed with the accompanying grasses, making it a very suitable species for grazing. It has the quality of being able to grow well in a wide variety of soils, except in non-calcareous and rough soils.

It has been observed that *Teramnus* associated with grasses has a good productive performance if rotations are made every 28-35 days in the rainy season and every 45 days in the dry season.

In cutting experiments, yields between 10-18 t/ha of DM have been reported, although it is more convenient to use it in rotational grazing.

Morus spp. (Mulberry)

This legume can also be used for livestock purposes and is a good option to produce forage. It adapts to any type of soil but prefers loose and well-drained soil.

For its good development, this plant requires chemical or organic fertilization that provides around 250 kg of N, 150 kg of P and 50 kg of K per year/ha, applied fractionally by cutting, especially nitrogen. It can produce between 50 and 60 t/ha of green forage per year (12-15 t/ha of DM).

In Cuba, yields of approximately 2 t/ha of DM/cut have been obtained during the dry season. In a mulberry plantation, the total biomass produced has an approximate composition of 45 % leaves, 5 % tender stems and 50 % woody stems.

Nutritional value

The dry matter content of the edible part ranges between 20 and 24 %. Mulberry is one of the legumes with the highest digestibility (80-90 %) and high crude protein content (17-25 %).

In cattle fed with grass and mulberry supplemented with feed, milk productions of over 12 kg/cow/day were achieved, and daily increases in live weight in calves between 600 and 620 g/animal.

Canavalia sp. (Canavalia bean)

This legume has high protein and energy values. There are more than 20 species of the *Canavalia genus*, but only three of them:

a) Ensiformis
b) Gladiate
c) Maritima

are suitable as animal feed due to their high protein content. Under direct grazing, these species can produce between two to three t/ha of DM and 0.5 t of crude protein.

As green fodder, pure fodder areas can be sown near the unit, or traditional fodder areas can be intercropped with Canavalia.

This legume can be processed as flour to include it in the manufacture of feed, drying and grinding its leaves that contain between 20 to 22 % protein.

Centrosema plumieri. (Centrosema ecotype Mayari)

This plant has shown good establishment when its seeds are spread at a rate of 6 kg/ha, on natural grass before or immediately after grazing in good soil moisture conditions. With this, the productivity of the pasture was increased by 26 % and its protein value.

Another way of using Centrosema is by intercropping it with temporary forage plants that serve as support, such as sorghum, corn, sunflower, kenaf, etc. When intercropped with sorghum, it can increase DM production by more than 2 t/ha and have up to 34 % participation in the production of total biomass.

Cajanus cajan. (Pigeon bean)

It is one of the most cultivated legumes in tropical areas. Due to its high nutritional value, it has been compared to alfalfa, but it has the difficulty of being unappetizing to livestock.

This shrub can produce 20-30 t/ha/DM of fodder with more than 18 % CP. It is quite resistant to drought, but only provides good yields with rainfall greater than 500 mm.

This plant is not very demanding in terms of soil but is more productive when sown in loose and deep soil.

Pigeon pea varieties are differentiated by the length of the vegetative period. The earliest ones mature in 3-5 months and have small seeds; the semi-late ones mature in 5-7 months, the late ones in 7-12 months and have large seeds.

Pigeon pea can be used to produce fodder mixed with other grasses. The plants cut at the time of flowering can be made into hay and even ensiled with good results.

Two harvests can be obtained per year. The seeds are used for human consumption and as feed for livestock. The green pods and leaves can constitute an excellent fodder.

Due to its high protein content, it can be associated with grasses established on savannah soils supported by serpentine soil, except those affected by excessive salinity or where there are floods.

Associations of grasses with legumes

The inclusion of legumes in any pasture exploitation system leads to notable benefits, because this type of plants has, in their roots, nodules with nitro-fixing bacteria that can take nitrogen from the air and enrich the soil with this element.

In addition, they are a safe source of high biological value proteins and other nutritional properties such as:

a) High percentage of crude protein (15-30 %)

b) High percentage of digestibility (58-60 %)

c) High content of vitamins (A, B, C and D)

d) They are rich in Ca, P, Mg and K

e) High amount of metabolizable energy (ME) (2,2-2,7 Mcal/kg of DM)

Due to all these benefits, its association with forage and grazing grasses favors obtaining a greater quantity of biomass per unit of area with a higher quality, especially due to the improvement of the protein-energy ratio.

Forage grasses

The best results have been obtained in associations of the grasses *Sorghum bicolor* (Grain sorghum, Forage sorghum), King grass and *Saccharum officinarum L.* (Sugar cane), with the climbing legumes *Centrosema plumieri* (Butterfly pea), *Stizolobium aterrimum* (Velvet bean or mucuna), *Neonotonia wightii* (Glycine) and *Clitoriaternatea* (Blue shell) among others.

Centrosema plumieri with *Sorghum bicolor*

Both crops are sown in the same furrow in a light stream, at a rate of 5 kg/ha for Sorghum and 3 kg/ha for Centrosema; the distance between furrows will be 0.70 m.

After 90 days, the harvest will be carried out, repeating the sowing of Centrosema in the furrow left after cultivating *Sorghum*.

The production of DM obtained with this practice, both in experimental plots and in production areas, has been higher than that achieved in both crops without association.

Stizolobium aterrimum. (Mucuna or Velvet) with ***Sorghum bicolor.*** (Sorghum)

This association exceeds the production of forage to pure crops or without association, doubling the yields per area of sorghum sown alone, highlighting that velvet provides practically a similar amount of forage to sorghum, without considering the 7 % of the spike existing in the total biomass.

***Stizolobium aterrimum* + *Sorghum bicolor* + King grass**

In King grass, being the most widespread forage variety in our livestock, is where the greatest productive impact could be obtained by systematically associating it with forage legumes.

This association doubles the percentage of CP of the biomass obtained. In association with forage sorghum, it increases DM yields by more than 3 t/ha, while improving the CP percentage by more than 5 %.

Grazing grasses

Considering the high dependence of our livestock on direct grazing in the field, together with the poor quality of the predominant natural pastures, which do not exceed 5 % in their CP content, the need to associate legumes with grazing grasses is understood.

The inclusion of *Crotalaria juncea* in natural pastures produces a notable improvement in production per area and in the quality of the biomass to be consumed by livestock.

Among the varieties of this species, *Crotalaria juncea* cv Nett is the one that has shown the best qualities to be used in associations with grazing grasses in Cuba.

Association with forage sugar cane

Due to its low protein content (2-3 %), it is forage sugar cane that most needs to be associated with legumes.

Legume varieties to be used

Macroptilium atropurpureum cv. *Siratro* and glycine (*Neonotonia wightii*) have been highlighted for association; however, other varieties that stand out locally should not be ruled out, considering regionalization and their possibilities for association.

In Holguín province, Cuba the associations obtained with *Centrosema plumieri* and the spontaneous associations frequently observed in plantations with *Teramnus labialis* were successful.

Conservation of pastures and forages

The conservation of pastures and forages in the form of hay and silage has long been an integral component of animal feeding systems in temperate zones of the world as a way of maintaining the supply of forage for high-production animals throughout the year.

However, its use in the tropics has been limited to small productions, generally of poor quality.

How can we explain its low use in countries that have a dry season that lasts six months or more?

This question can be analyzed from different aspects, but the main ones are not having forage areas, lack of material resources, lack of knowledge of technologies, shortage of labor and little perception of the risk of drought.

Another aspect that has threatened the conservation of forage is that mowing must be done during the rainiest season and the waters hinder the production of hay or silage.

This is true, but if the weather forecast services provided by the Provincial Meteorological Stations were used, the harmful effects of the waters during the process could be minimized.

Currently these stations make short-term weather forecasts and can predict three to five days in advance whether it will rain or not in each region.

Haymaking

The objective of haymaking is to reduce the water content of green fodder to less than 20 % so that it can be stored in large quantities without severe fermentation or mold.

The process must be carried out in such a way that the fodder does not discolor, does not lose its nutrients, and keeps leaf loss to a minimum.

Good quality hay is obtained by cutting plants at a suitable stage of maturity, with abundant leaves, soft and pliable stems, a green or light brown color and few foreign materials, free of molds, and having the typical fragrance of the crop from which it is made.

The main mistakes made in hay production are: cutting the grass when the stems are lignified and have few leaves, exposing them to the sun for many days and storing them in inappropriate places. The result of this procedure is a product of poor nutritional quality, closer to straw than to real hay.

To avoid these errors, the age of cutting the grass should be between 6 and 9 weeks, in a vegetative state or beginning to spike (40 and 45 days), however, the development of the plant should be considered regardless of age.

The radio information provided by the Weather Forecast Department of the Provincial Meteorological Stations should be sought, to select the most propitious days for mowing and drying the forage and not exposing it to the sun for more than three days.

Good hay can be produced from almost all the species and varieties of regionalized grasses and legumes mentioned in this chapter, if the correct technology is applied and it is kept in suitable haylofts.

The latter must be considered since the conservation of hay in the humid tropics has an important limiting factor with the high relative humidity of the air, which persists throughout the year. Dark and poorly ventilated haylofts encourage the deterioration of hay due to the action of fungi.

Dehydration and grinding of tree plants

Flours obtained from the dehydration and grinding of tree foliage have been used as a protein component of nutritional blocks with good results in replacing concentrates or as a supplementary feed.

Advantages of preserving food in the form of flour

Its structure allows its inclusion in a wide variety of foods.

It facilitates the storage of food for long periods.

The manufacture of flour can help improve the consumption of biomass produced by some trees that are not very tasty when fresh.

The high protein content means that flours can be used as a protein supplement combined with other raw materials or partially replacing cereal concentrates.

Actions for flour production

The production of flour from tree plants such as *Leucaena leucocephala, Albizia lebbeck, Gliricidia sepium, Morus alba* and *Moringa oleifera* involves a group of activities that are not usual in livestock systems, such as:

a) Establishing forage areas for the legumes.

b) Drying in the sun.

c) Grinding and mixing with 3-5 % cane molasses to make it more palatable to animals.

Tree plant flour can be used as a partial substitute for cereal concentrates or together with other supplementation components.

Silage

Conservation in the form of silage is a technique that has very precise rules. Failure to apply them properly affects the quality of the product and the farmer's confidence. Without forage with good nutritional value, satisfactory silage cannot be achieved.

How to achieve the best quality of forage for conservation?

There are two aspects to consider: age and quality. If age increases, quality decreases, expressed by nutritional value (protein and digestibility), but the volume to be conserved increases.

The so-called grazing species, in practical terms, have the acceptable value for ensiling between 6 and 7 weeks and forage species between 9 and 10 weeks.

Fertilization has a significant effect on yield and crude protein content, but not on nutrient digestibility and consumption.

The optimal levels are around 60 kg of N/ha/cut and are recommended to obtain good yields and adequate quality.

Conservation must be carried out with the minimum loss of nutrients and ensiled material.

To meet these requirements, the following factors must be observed:

a) Particle size and chopping
b) Manufacturing time
c) Compaction
d) Height
e) Additives
f) Covering

It is important to build the silo near the dairy farm, in a high place to facilitate natural drainage.

The literature describes numerous ways of building a silo, which depends on the resources available to the farmer.

For small producers, the most convenient silos are those of small dimensions, no larger than two tons, which allow all manipulations to be done in one day, without the need for compaction of mechanized implements.

There are different variants, such as: mixed silages in plastic bags or using ring silos.

In practice, rectangular trench silos, with a capacity of 2 m^3, are the most used and their acceptance lies in the fact that they are easy to adapt to the specific conditions of each farm. Its vulnerable aspects are the need to achieve adequate hermeticity and that there is a balance between the dimensions of the silo and the volume of forage to be conserved.

Characteristics that indicate the quality of silages

The qualitative indicators to consider are smell, color, texture and degree of humidity. If the silage has an olive green color, it is considered excellent; if it is yellowish green, it is good.

The smell must be pleasant, like ripe fruit or wine. A pleasant and light smell of vinegar is allowed. It should not leave residue on the hands when touched. As for texture, the leaves must remain attached to the stem and the hairs of the fresh grass must be observed. When it is taken, it should not wet the hands, and the material should be kept loose.

If the silage is brown or almost black, with a putrid or rancid smell, if the texture is soapy to the touch, if it exudes liquids when taken, we are in the presence of a poor-quality silage.

What forages can be ensiled?

Corn is unsurpassed for its conditions to form good silage. Cut when all its leaves are still green, but the grain has already formed (beginning of hardening after the dough stage), it has a high yield (more than 25 tons per hectare) and a considerably high nutrient content (18 to 20 % on a wet basis). Its juicy, full stems and broad, soft leaves allow for uniform and easy compaction. But there are many other plants that can be successfully ensiled. In fact, if certain precautions are taken, almost any green forage can be ensiled.

In sugar cane producing countries, the cane tips or buds that are abundant during the sugar harvest can be used to make silage of acceptable quality. Because of its free sugar content, this silage does not require additives. However, when the tips are very dry, the resulting silage is of very poor quality.

Precautions for successful ensiling

Do not use forage that is too hard or has hollow stems that make compaction difficult, chop the forage to less than 2 cm, do not use forage with more than 25 % dry matter.

Success in ensiling is also ensured by adding diluted cane molasses as a preservative, when required.

Haylage

It is an intermediate product between silage and hay, where the percentage of dry matter achieved with pre-drying is approximately 50 %. The quality of this product tends to be more stable than silage, if it is processed properly. This form of forage conservation has been used for years by cattle breeders in Brazil, Mexico and other Central American countries.

Limitations of the use of standards in dairy cattle

In Livestock Nutrition and Dietetics, it is indicated that *"the food balance is carried out considering the food available to the unit. The energy, protein and mineral requirements for each category and animal group are evaluated. In case there is a deficit, it must be determined how to compensate for it"*.

These indications can be fulfilled when balanced rations are administered, but not when dealing with cows in pastures.

It is natural that in practice it is not known how much forage a grazing animal eats, and much less the dry matter content or composition of it. Furthermore, in the case of stabled animals it is not customary to weigh the silage or green forage that is given to each cow.

We can therefore conclude that in practice a dairy ration is never fully balanced according to the requirements suggested by the standards.

How then can the practical farmer guide himself in feeding his cows?

It is obvious that bulky fodder, whether hay, cut fodder, silage or grazing, must be supplied at will and to all his cows on equal terms.

He can divide the herd into high and low producers and give the best fodder or grazing to the high producers.

From then on there is only one course to take and that is to try to find out how deficient the bulky fodder is in meeting the nutritional requirements of the animal.

This is especially important in the dry season when grasses practically disappear from the pastures.

The first indication of nutritional imbalance is the reduction of milk production.

Any milk production obtainable from such a cow would have to be at the expense of her tissues, i.e. by losing body mass.

Thus, by simply observing the state of the animal's flesh, it is possible to know if the feed received meets the production or maintenance requirements.

In practice, I have observed how the farmer is content with offering the animal a third of what it needs in its daily ration and does not comply with the standard of 25 kg of bulky feed required.

Hence the importance of the technical or professional staff who care for the herd being concerned about the quality and quantity of bulky feed provided to the animals each day, especially during the dry period. In this case, the best balance is the productive and physical response of the animal to the diet it is receiving.

Contribution of agroforestry to food self-sufficiency

Due to logging, burning and the use of concrete or dry wood posts for fences, the grazing areas of most farms and livestock farms in tropical countries do not have adequate natural tree shade, nor can they use trees as sources of feed for livestock.

In addition, the quality and productivity of pastures has been reduced due to increased evapotranspiration, erosion and inadequate grazing methods.

In all tropical countries there should be laws that encourage, support and encourage livestock farm owners to use living fences and other silvipastoral procedures to protect soil and animals.

From the point of view of the practices they comprise and their functions, silvipastoral systems can be classified as: protein banks, associations of trees with pastures, living fences and windbreaks.

Protein banks

In livestock farming, protein banks are the areas of dense and compact sowing with plants with a high protein content (generally legumes) that are subjected to directed grazing.

The system consists of sowing trees, shrubs and creeping herbaceous legumes in combination or not with grasses, at high densities, in a portion of the grazing area (between 20 and 30 % of the area), with the aim of being used as a protein supplement, mainly in times of food shortage.

The most common is to use perennial plants, either creeping plants such as Glycine, *Centrosema* or *Teramnus* or trees such as Leucaena and Moringa. The association of climbing legumes with trees allows for a greater amount of biomass per unit area, by enveloping the primary stems of trees, which are generally leafless.

Associations of trees with pastures

The systems of association of trees with pastures are called silvipastoral because they establish a harmonious relationship between them, based on the well-being of farm animals and biodiversity.

The animals graze throughout the grazing area and in turn consume the leaves, fruits, bark and other parts of the trees. The presence of trees in pastures also provides shade and shelter for livestock.

The use of leguminous trees in these systems also helps to rehabilitate soils through a strong recirculation of nutrients and the symbiotic fixation of N.

This last characteristic of the association gives it advantages over Protein Bank systems, which cannot be used as soil contributors and improvers, since only 20 to 30 % of the total area is devoted to trees.

Environmental services

The presence of trees affects water dynamics by acting as a barrier that controls runoff; as cover, reducing the impact of water drops; and as soil improvers, increasing infiltration and water retention.

Carbon sequestration

Agroforestry systems have two main benefits for carbon conservation:

1) Direct storage of C in the short and medium term (decades or centuries) in trees and soil.

2) Direct reduction of greenhouse gas emissions caused by deforestation and shifting agriculture.

In the different silvipastoral systems, the production and extraction of wood for construction, firewood, charcoal, poles, etc., can reduce the pressure on natural resources in forests and fossil fuels, so there is an indirect positive impact on C conservation in other ecosystems.

Another advantage is that silvipastoral systems, with their dispersed trees, do not allow the burning of pastures, which is another source of CO_2 emissions, which is still used in some countries in the regeneration of pastures.

Depending on the topographic and relief characteristics of the grazing areas, tree planting can be done in different ways: trees in compact stands, trees in pastures for shade, scattered trees or in groups, trees in contours (living fences and windbreaks), trees in alleys and corners.

The most important thing is that the species selected are regionalized, are mostly legumes and that biodiversity is considered, that is, interspersing trees of different species, whether forage, timber, honey or fruit.

Regionalization of trees to improve ecosystems

Like pastures, trees do not have the same behavior in different soil and climate conditions, with some performing better than others in certain livestock ecosystems; Leucaena, for example, grows poorly in low soils prone to waterlogging, while Blackbead or Manila tamarind (*Pithecelobium dulce*) with similar forage aptitudes, adapts perfectly to these.

Based on surveys of producers and inventories of tree species adapted to different ecosystems, the Holguín Pasture and Forage Experimental Station proposed planting trees with Siris Tree, White Mulberry, Mountain Ebony, Quickstick, Manila Tamarind, White Lead Tree, Rain Tree, Coral Tree, Bastard Cedar, and Pigeon Pea in the different livestock ecosystems of that province, to use them in silvipastoral systems. See the nutritional characteristics of these plants in the following table.

The forage species that have performed best in silvipastoral systems are:

Gliricidia sepium, Erythrina spp, Erythrina glauca, Erythrina americana, Guazuma ulmifolia, Alcalypha tenicu caudata, Leucaena leucocephala, Diphysa robinioides, Trichanthera gigantea and *Tithonia diversifolia.*

Table 1-1 shows the chemical composition and nutritional properties of the trees that adapt well to the conditions of the tropic.

Table 1-1 Chemical composition and digestibility of trees recommended by EEPF Holguin

Common name	Scientific name	CP	Ca	P	DM%
Siris Tree	Albizia lebbeck	20	2,00	0,15	65
White Mulberry	Morus alba	22	2,40	0,24	87
Mountain Ebony	Bauhinia variegata L.	16	1,75	0,18	56
Quickstick	Gliricidia sepium	26	1,70	0,27	66
Manila Tamarind	Pithecelobium dulce	22	1,60	0,31	67
White Leadtree	L. leucocephala	25	1,54	0,29	65
Rain Tree	Pithecellobium saman	25	1,00	0,23	66
Coral Tree	Erythrina Spp	21	1,00	0,23	60
Bastard Cedar	Guazuma tomentosa	17	1,33	0,24	57
Pigeon Pea	Cajanus cajan	26	1,72	0,24	59

Legend: CP = crude protein; DM = dray matter

Living fences and windbreaks

A living fence is a line of trees or bushes that delimit an environment; but it can be used as a provider of animal feed in emergency situations.

In Cuba, legumes, shrubs or small trees have been used, with the capacity to sprout and be reproduced by cuttings. In addition, those with multiple uses are more frequently selected, capable of providing wood for direct use, firewood, fodder, or that are melliferous or medicinal.

Among the most used species are: *Erythrina berteroana, Echinodorus grisebachii* (Amazon sword plant), *E. poeppigiana, Gliricidia sepium* (Quickstick), *Jatropha curcas* (Nutmeg plant).

In addition, other non-leguminous tree species have been used such as: *Bursera simaruba* (Gumbo-limbo) for its easy reproduction by cuttings and for its medicinal use, *Guazuma ulmifolia* (Bay cedar), *Pithecellobium* sweet, *Spondias mombin* (Yellow mombin), *Spondias sp* (Hog plums) for the ease with which they are propagated by cuttings and because their fruits are eaten by pigs and cattle.

The simplest way to make a living fence and to have enough propagules is the following: hardwood logs are buried in rows every 10 meters to serve as support for the smooth or barbed wire threads.

Green stakes are obtained from sturdy branches no less than two meters long and a sharp beveled point is made at one end. To bury them more easily, holes 20-25 cm deep are made with a crowbar and they are planted in rows one meter apart.

The wire threads are fixed to the green stakes with henequen ropes or other material, so as not to damage their bark. The wire must be fixed with metal staples after the first year of growth of the stake.

Table 1-2 shows the results of the utilitarian value of the main fodder trees used in Latin America. Note that *Erythrina berteroana, Erythrina poeppigiana, Gliricidia sepium, Leucaena leucocephala* and *Moringa oleifera* were the most integral since they can be used as living fences, as shade and for feeding cattle, goats, sheep and rabbits. Almost all of them can be used as living hedges.

Table 1-2 Utility value of fodder trees

Species: botanical name	1	2	3	4	5	6	7
Acacia farnesiana						x	
Aralia sp	x	x	x				
Bambusa vulgaris		x	x			x	x
Bursera simaruba	x	x					
Citrus spp	x		x			x	x
Dichrostachys glomerata						x	
Erythrina berteroana	x	x	x			x	x
Erythrina poeppigiana	x	x	x			x	x
Gliricidia sepium	x	x	x			x	x
Jatropha curcas	x	x					
Leucaena leucocephala	x	x	x	x	x	x	x
Moringa oleifera	x	x	x			x	x
Persea americana	x		x				
Spondias purpurea	x	x					
Trichanthera gigantea	x		x	x			
Trichilia hirta	x	x					

Legend: Numbers represent possible uses:
1- For shade.
2- For living fences.
3- For cattle feed.
4- For sheep feed.
5- For rabbit feed.
6- For goat feed.
7- For pig feed.

On the other hand, and although they are not forest species, farmers use *Bromelia pinguin* (Wild pineapple), which in some cases constitutes barriers to stop erosion, and *Lemaireocereus hystrix* (Cardona), a species of cactus, as living hedges.

A windbreak consists of lines of trees (from one to three) that protect a field of pastures, crops or trees from the harmful action of the strong trade winds that blow regularly from the northeast and the north, which can reach up to 100 km/h and the dry winds from the south, up to 126 km/h, but less frequent, and from tropical storms and cyclones that sometimes hit tropical regions.

A windbreak can also be a living fence, or vice versa. The use of these systems is a widely used practice in Central America and the Caribbean, since living fences not only serve as support for wire fences, but also produce products such as fruit, fodder, firewood, wood, flowers for honey, posts, etc.

Additionally, the use of living fences represents a saving for the rancher, since durable wooden posts and concrete posts have reached prohibitive prices.

In addition to the species mentioned for living fences, *Callophyllum brasiliense* (Brazil Beauty-Leaf), *Casuarina equisetifolia* (Coastal she-oak), *Citrus limon*, *Eucalyptus saligna* (Sydney Blue Gum), *Hibiscus elatus* (Blue mahoe), and *Tamarix indica* (Tamarisk), *Mangifera indica* (Mango), can be included, with the exception that they must be planted in seedlings.

Biodiversity conservation

The accelerated deforestation and burning of forests to convert them into crop and pasture areas that has occurred and is occurring in many countries, especially in South America (Amazon) and Africa, seriously affects the survival of many plant and animal species. For one of these reasons, living fences can help in their conservation.

The connection of different boundaries in the form of a corridor influences the movement of animals and the dispersion of plants. Birds of different species use trees as habitat and are the most important vectors for the dissemination of seeds.

It must be recognized that living hedges are a complex ecological system due to their diversity. They constitute contact zones between groups of species typical of the natural environment and agriculture.

In hedges there are 20 species of grasses, 10-15 of shrubs, and three to seven of trees. They are the point of convergence of two ecosystems (the forest and the field), where the richness of animal and plant species is high.

In addition, hedgerows encourage the concentration of a wide variety of insectivorous bird species: in all seasons of the year, which consume large quantities of insects and larvae. In this way, birds become active elements in pest control.

Results of the introduction of the silvipastoral system in livestock farms

Silvipastoral systems began to be developed in the 1980s, based on studies carried out by agricultural research centers in the country.

Over the last 35 years, a large amount of important scientific information has been accumulated, sufficient to improve the food situation of Cuban livestock.

As an example, I inform you of some reproductive and productive results that have been obtained with the establishment of silvipastoral systems in different provinces of Cuba.

From a reproductive point of view, with the introduction of silvipastoral systems, in several herds of Siboney cows in the province of Villa Clara, an ICFI of 111 ± 24 and 103.6 ± 38 days, an ICC of 172.8 ± 38 and 147.3 ± 24 days and an CI of 454.2 ± 38 and 427.3 ± 25 days was achieved, 1.9 and 2.1 services were needed per conception.

In a herd of 958 purebred Criollo cows, with a total of 2,745 births in ten years, an average age at incorporation of 23 ± 5.4 months was obtained; a weight at incorporation of 310.3 ± 21 kg; age at first calving 37.8 ± 11.4 months; ICFI 124.4 ± 84 days; ICC 175.4±98.8 days; PR 1.64±0.8.

On a livestock farm in Matanzas, in Holstein heifers, an average age at incorporation into reproduction of 22.3±1 month was achieved with a body mass of 304.5±3.2 kg; an age at gestation of 24.1±2 months and an average age at first calving of 33 months.

From the productive point of view, the rational management of the soil-pasture-animal-tree complex allowed the production of between 2,000 and 5,000 kg of milk/ha/year and has made it possible to obtain average daily gains close to 700 g day, with a final weight between 400 and 445 kg and yields of 800 kg of meat on the hoof/ha/year in crossbred fattening cattle.

Body mass increases of between 450 g/a-day and 600 g/animal-day have also been achieved in the rearing of replacement females, with a weight of 290-300 kg at 24-27 months of age.

Conditions for planting trees in livestock systems

On many farms and ranches where trees are very scarce, farmers may not be willing to grow them. Traditionally, many attempts to replace complex traditional land use systems have failed, apparently due to the risks of climate, pests, difficulties in soil management and social and cultural conditions that hinder the acceptance of new systems.

According to FAO (1988) the main conditions that must be met before farmer's plant trees in their breeding systems are:

1) **Economic:** There must be sufficient land, seed, capital and labor resources available to make tree cultivation possible and to cover the costs of planting, caring for, harvesting and marketing them and their products. There is often a shortage of plants, a lack of quality control in the production of seeds and seedlings, a lack of information on propagation techniques, a lack of incentives and adequate credits for tree planting, all of this linked to the lack of adequate technical dissemination.

2) **Sociocultural:** The changes that tree cultivation may bring about in terms of productivity relationships and resource ownership models must be framed within culturally accepted strategies for resource distribution. The social value of trees must coincide with the values that the management measures and interventions adopted may impose.

Among the socioeconomic and cultural benefits provided using agroforestry practices, we can mention the reduction of economic risks for the rancher by achieving the diversification of production, the use of family labor with a better integration of family members into the production process, and the maintenance of customs or practices of land use, which are deeply rooted in culture, in some cases.

3) **Environmental:** Interventions or adaptation efforts must consider adequate knowledge of the conditions of the chosen sites, the availability of water, the temperature regime, as well as other characteristics of the natural environment.

These conditions may include some factors that limit or make impossible the planting of trees on livestock farms in the tropics.

a) The livestock tradition of the producer

Extensive livestock management is the work that they know best and know best how to do, therefore, the adoption of agrosilvipastoral techniques for the rancher is more difficult, due in large part to their lack of knowledge.

b) Availability of labor

Most agrosilvipastoral techniques require different management for each of the established components. The periods of use and the amount of labor, generally expensive and scarce, are important in the decision of whether to adopt the proposed alternatives.

c) Land use management plan

Not all farms are susceptible to being used in agrosilvipastoral arrangements due to the costs involved and the natural differences that make up the microclimates. It is therefore necessary, over time, to determine and define the most suitable areas for each component, considering factors such as soil quality, topography, previous use, ease of access and others that are considered important in the success of the company.

Chapter 2

Effects of tropical climate on animal economy

Contents:
Introduction. Tropical climate as a limiting factor. Direct effects of climate on cattle. General characteristics of tropical climate. Environmental stress in animals. Relationships between heat tolerance and heat stress. How to prevent or mitigate the harmful effects of environmental stress and drought. Soil and its conservation.

Introduction

The direct effects of climatic elements on the morphological, physiological, productive and reproductive characteristics of cattle have been reliably proven at all latitudes. Climatic influences are even greater if the indirect effects on the other components of the livestock agroecosystem are included, particularly through pastures and forage, soils and other living elements that exist in this particular type of ecosystem.

Tropical climate as a limiting factor

The effects of tropical climate on livestock and other living components of the agro-ecosystem are similar to those of other environmental factors and are in accordance with the ecological law of Limiting Factors, which indicates the limiting effect that can be presented on the subsistence, development or productive or reproductive behavior of any living organism or population by those environmental factors that are, to a greater or lesser extent, above or below the maximum or minimum tolerance level of the species, also known as the Law of Maximum and Law of Minimum, respectively.

The existence of this law is closely related to the so-called Shelford Law of Tolerance, which describes that for each biological process of an organism there will be a maximum and a minimum lethal limit, outside of which the process ceases or leads to the death of the organism.

An optimal range can also be distinguished, within which the process achieves its best results. The maximum and minimum lethal values, as well as the optimal range, will depend on the genetic characteristics of the organism or population, varying between species, races and even between individuals, and even within the same individual.

Direct effects of climate in cattle

Climate is defined as the characteristic physical state of the atmosphere of a given place on the earth's surface over a long period of years. Its momentary situation is known as the weather. Both depend on the gaseous composition of the atmosphere and the physical processes that take place in it.

Given its condition as a dynamic system, the structure and functioning of the climate will be determined not only by the individual variation of each of its component elements, but also by the links and interactions between them, that is, by the structure and function of the whole.

For example, solar radiation determines the warming of the earth's surface by influencing the temperature of the earth. This in turn warms the atmosphere by causing the temperature of the air to vary. The energy supplied directly by solar radiation or indirectly by the air or the earth allows evaporation, the accumulation of air humidity and later, by cooling, condensation and precipitation to take place. In turn, differences in the temperatures of different areas of the earth's surface will cause inverse variations in atmospheric pressure, and these differences determine the movement of air masses parallel to said surface from high pressure areas to low pressure areas, generating the meteorological phenomenon known as wind.

The gaseous composition of the atmosphere, its vertical distribution and various meteorological elements, especially those related to the hydrological cycle, play a regulatory role within the system, influencing the greater or lesser reflection and absorption of solar energy, and therefore the energy that naturally enters agricultural systems and their heating.

Of these climate elements, air temperature, solar radiation, humidity, wind and precipitation are those that have the most marked effect on cattle, especially dairy breeds.

Each of these elements acts as a subsystem composed of different variables, closely interrelated with each other, as we will see below.

General characteristics of the tropical climate

The effective use of the climate as a natural resource and the protection of the environment require that we know its main characteristics, its variations and the changes that occur in it, as well as the relationship between these variations and the different components of the environment.

According to the influence of marine currents and other geographic peculiarities, the following types of climates have been proposed:

1) **Relatively dry tropical.**

2) **Relatively humid tropical.** Which is the one that predominates in its spatial distribution and characterizes the plains, except those of the dry tropics.

3) **Humid tropical.** With rain almost all year round and which is associated with mountain systems between 200 and 500 m high.

4) **Warm temperate.** With rain almost all year round, which occupies mountainous territories at more than 500 m high.

Air temperature

This is the climatic element that most directly influences cattle. Its values determine the effect of solar radiation, wind and humidity, whose combined action on animals will depend on the thermal state of the air.

The main variables that characterize this element are the mean temperature, mean minimum temperature and mean maximum temperature, and the difference between the last two is known as thermal amplitude or oscillation.

Although the maximum air temperature during the day is high, during the night it rarely exceeds 27 °C, which offers favorable conditions for cattle during the night period. In such conditions the animal can adapt to carry out its vital activities (such as grazing) during the night period.

During the day, if there is not much cloud cover, in all months of the year there are at least two hours of light thermal stress, which is noticeable during almost the entire daytime period from May to October. Monthly averages of maximum temperatures exceed the limit of 27 °C, indicated as the upper critical temperature for well-being in *Bos taurus* cattle.

It should be noted that, due to the time required for cooling and warming, there is a delay in the seasons. This delay is the result of a relaxation period between action and effect. For this reason, the warmest months are June, July and August and not May, June and July, and the coldest months are December, January and February instead of November, December and January as would be expected due to the amount of incident solar radiation and the date of the solstices.

Solar radiation

The tropical geographic zone benefits from a high incidence of solar radiation. Each square meter of tropical territory receives, on average annually, 5 kWh of solar energy daily. This energy is manifested in all regions of the electromagnetic spectrum, from gamma rays to ultraviolet radiation, passing through the visible zone, up to the infrared. Radiant energy that arrives directly from the Sun, without being interfered with by obstacles in its atmospheric path, is direct radiation. Radiation that is scattered, diffracted or reflected by particles suspended in the atmosphere constitutes diffuse radiation, including radiation reflected by clouds towards the earth.

The amount of radiation that is reflected under the same angle of incidence depends on the characteristics of the surface on which it falls. Light-colored surfaces reflect more and absorb less radiation, while dark surfaces do the opposite. The reflecting capacity of a surface is called albedo, which is the ratio between the reflected radiation and the summary radiation, which is the sum of direct and diffuse solar radiation. It is important to know that the albedo capacity of reservoir water is 80-85 %, that of pastures is 30-32 %, while that of forests is only 5-10 %.

Solar radiation is, after air temperature, the climate element with the greatest direct effect in cattle. It represents the contribution of radiant heat that reaches the animal through this route with a load that is generally excessive for its thermoregulatory mechanisms. Its annual range and the duration of the period of direct solar radiation are known as *insolation*.

The period of direct solar radiation is 7,2 hours and 5,1 hours, averages for February and October respectively. Considering that the milk and meat production system used in tropical countries is based on pastures, the animals must remain in pastures devoid of trees for most of the day, receiving direct solar radiation which, as will be seen later, noticeably accentuates the effects of environmental heat stress.

The maximum insolation in April (9,7 hours) coincides with the minimum cloudiness. The high cloudiness recorded in the warm-rainy period from May to October attenuates the effect of direct solar radiation during these months and determines that the proportion of diffuse radiation is, as an annual average, nationally, around 45 % of the total solar radiation.

The fact that solar radiation is more intense during the dry season worsens the water shortage situation, since it increases water evaporation, which further dries out reservoirs and pastures.

Relative humidity of the air

One of the characteristics of the tropical climate is that it has high atmospheric humidity throughout the year. The relative humidity of the air (RH) in the rainiest period is 82 % on average and 77 % in the less rainy period, with an annual average of 79 %.

The presence of a greater quantity of water vapor in the air contributes to altering the content of solar radiation since this vapor has a greater absorbing power of infrared radiation than air, which causes humid air to heat up more than dry air.

This high RH of the air directly influences the thermoregulation of cattle. It acts together with high temperatures and hinders the dissipation of heat from the animal through the most effective physical route in these thermal conditions: **evaporation**. Heat losses through this route depend on the gradient of water vapor tension of the skin or lung surface with respect to the surrounding air.

On the other hand, the high RH of the Cuban subtropical climate constitutes an important limiting factor in the conservation of food, particularly in the production and conservation of hay.

Wind

Wind is the mass movement of air in the atmosphere. It is also defined as "the compensation of atmospheric pressure differences between two points." According to their strength and direction, meteorologists classify them as gusts, squalls, breezes, gales, storms and hurricanes. The ascending or descending movement of air is called a current.

The effect of the wind favors the dissipation of heat from the animal when the temperature and water vapor tension of the air are higher than those of the animal's skin surface, so the temperature assumes the predominant role in relation to the effect of the wind.

If the air temperature is lower than the animal's comfort zone, the effect of the wind is harmful because it leads to excessive cooling of the animal (hypothermia). At moderately high temperatures or within the comfort zone, the wind favors the dissipation of heat by the cooling effect of evaporation.

However, if the air temperature continues to rise and approaches or exceeds skin temperature (33 °C), the effect can be harmful, since in such conditions the heat flow passes from the air to the animal.

It has been observed that the most favorable wind speeds for the normal growth and development of plants and animals are between 0.5 and 2 m/s. Stronger winds act unfavorably in animals and plants, depending on their intensity and duration.

The harmful effects of wind can be countered by building dense living fences and windbreaks, composed of one or several rows of trees and bushes in a direction perpendicular to the prevailing wind of the area.

These curtains can even protect livestock areas from the effects of dry southern winds and storms and cyclones that may penetrate the national territory.

Calm days

The unfavorable behavior of the wind regime in some tropical countries in relation to livestock is noteworthy, since the minimum values are found in the summer, when the effect of the wind is most beneficial, and decrease in September and October to values below 2 m/s.

During this hot period, calm days are very frequent, when the air barely moves and causes an increase in the respiratory rate of cattle.

Precipitation

The amount of precipitation determines the name given to the rainy and less rainy periods of the year. It can be said that precipitation is the most variable element of the climate of the tropics, both in spatial and temporal order.

However, there are some regularities in its distribution given the increase in precipitation on the coasts towards the interior and at the height above sea level.

In the inter-annual distribution of rainfall, a rainy period is distinguished with 80 % of the annual amount and a less rainy period with 20 %.

In the rainiest period, precipitation varies considerably in the plains from less than 400 mm on the coast, to 1 400 mm in the interior plains. In the mountain systems, values higher than 1 600 mm can be recorded.

From the end of June to October, hydrometeorological phenomena, particularly troughs and tropical waves, contribute significant amounts of rain to the water table and to the filling of reservoirs and dams.

Troughs, waves, tropical storms and hurricanes are often described as "*bad weather*" due to the local damage they can cause. However, it is these phenomena that provide the agroecosystem with the richest, most precious and essential element for life on earth: free water. Therefore, tropical hydrometeorological phenomena are essential to maintain the ecological balance of countries in tropical regions.

The dry season is characterized by relative homogeneity in the plains, with rainfall of the order of 350 to 250 mm and even less on different coasts.

The increase in rainfall at high altitudes is notable, particularly in the mountains, where levels exceeding 1,000 mm are recorded in the period from November to April.

In general, June is the rainiest month, with a secondary maximum in October. The lowest rainfall occurs in February.

Since the rains of the less rainy period come from cold fronts, the greater or lesser abundance of rainfall will depend on the number of cold fronts that penetrate the area.

Drought

Rain is of vital agricultural importance in the tropics. It replenishes the surface and deep-water table and maintains the flow of rivers and reservoirs.

Precipitation has its greatest effect on cattle indirectly, through the growth of grass and forage, which promotes and increases the availability of bulky food.

The direct effects of rain are also important and noticeable. Rain, falling directly on the animal, dissipates body heat by conduction and contributes to its cooling. The water retained in the coat, when subsequently evaporated, also causes the same effect.

Drought can be defined as a temporary anomaly in which the availability of water falls below the statistical requirements of a given geographical area. There is not enough *water* to supply the needs of plants, animals and humans.

The main cause of all droughts is the lack of rain, and this phenomenon is called ***meteorological drought***. If it persists, it leads to a ***hydrological drought***, characterized by the inequality between the natural availability of water and the natural demands for water.

Hydrological drought is related to the availability of water on the surface and below it, and is not usually simultaneous with the others, but occurs after meteorological or agricultural drought and can continue even after the other droughts have disappeared.

The 20 % of annual precipitation that falls in the least rainy period is not enough to supply the water requirements of natural and cultivated pastures and leads to ***livestock drought***, in which lignification and drying of pastures occur, which severely affects the availability of food for livestock.

The lack of water for a prolonged period causes *agricultural drought*, which limits or prevents the development of crops in general. Therefore, from an agricultural point of view, it is not incorrect to classify this period as dry.

Seasonal droughts are most common in the months that end the winter season, mainly March, April and May, when the heat increases, and the summer rains do not arrive. The process generally damages larger areas of land than floods and sometimes leads to real natural disasters.

It is known that the drought phenomenon is a normal component of climate variability, ENSO events and others, but it can also be a consequence of climate changes that have been occurring worldwide.

The Cuban Institute of Meteorology predicts temperature increases of between 1.6 and 2.5 °C by 2100, which will determine an increase in evaporation that will favor aridity. There will be an uncertain behavior of precipitation and a probable increase in droughts and sea level.

Livestock farmers must prepare to face the effects of drought through the agro-silvipastoral procedures already discussed in Chapter 1 and maintain constant vigilance for early warnings and forecasts that contribute to timely action.

To do so, they can use the Climate Monitoring Bulletin, provided by the Early Warning Systems of the provincial Meteorological Centers, with monthly and annual output.

Microclimate

From an ecological point of view, it is a local climate with characteristics different from those of the area in which it is located. It can also be defined as a set of atmospheric conditions that characterize a small environment or area.

The factors that make up a microclimate are topography, temperature, humidity, altitude-latitude, light and plant cover. This local climate that characterizes a small environment refers to geographic areas of tens of km^2 in size.

However, from a biological and zootechnical point of view, the microclimate must be conceptualized by paying more attention to the living space in which animals are raised. For example, the microclimate of a sow is its pigsty. That of a herd of cows is the environment of the farm or ranch.

Environmental stress in animals

Environmental stress breaks the balance of an organism, that is, its homeostatic state, as a consequence of the action of a negative stimulus coming from outside or inside the organism, which is called a stressor.

In response to this stimulus, a series of behavioral and physiological reactions are triggered in order to adapt as best as possible to this new situation. In this response, the organism activates its hypothalamus-sympathetic-chromaffin axis and the hypothalamus-pituitary-adrenal axis.

Endorphins, which are opioid neurotransmitters produced in the Central Nervous System, act as modulators of pain, body temperature, hunger and reproductive functions, and participate in the physiological mechanism of stress. In the face of a continued aggressive agent, endorphins, especially β-endorphin, act by stimulating the anterior pituitary gland to release ACTH. This hormone stimulates the adrenal glands to secrete corticosteroids, which help the organism to confront the aggression.

From a physiological point of view, this reaction is beneficial for the animal since it allows it to recover its previously altered homeostatic state.

If this situation becomes chronic, the animal no longer has the capacity to react and this creates problems in the growth, reproductive, osmo-regulatory and immune processes that are reflected at the level of the organism and the herd.

In tropical environmental conditions, the main stressors for cattle are heat, chronic malnutrition and lack of water.

Heat stress

When the animal exceeds the upper limit of the thermoneutral zone, maintaining its normal body temperature begins to alter its basal metabolic rate. The combined effect of high temperatures, RH and low wind speed, especially when the animal grazes in the bright sun, generates a state of physiological and behavioral responses that affect its normal state of well-being.

The repercussions of heat stress are influenced by a series of adaptation mechanisms of the organism itself.

But the fact is that it temporarily affects: the animal's productivity, reproductive fitness and health.

The best-known harmful effects of heat stress on the reproduction of dairy cows are shortened duration of heat and its expression, repeated services, early embryonic mortality, decreased uterine blood flow, dysfunction of the corpus luteum, all of which lead to decreased fertility.

In general, heat stress causes a decrease in feed consumption and milk production, particularly in dairy cows of European breeds that have a less effective heat tolerance.

Relationships between heat tolerance and heat stress

Heat tolerance is a vital requirement for bovine livestock production in the tropics. It is defined as the individual's ability to efficiently use energy without generating excessive heat, maintaining its productivity at high levels.

It is measured through the tolerance index and when an animal has 100 it is considered well adapted to the ambient temperature and humidity. *Critical points* have been established where the ambient temperature causes physiological reactions of metabolic activity in bovines.

First critical point

Is thermo-neutrality, which corresponds to the ambient temperature at which body heat is in equilibrium.

Second critical point

Is the range of ambient temperature between 6 °C and 21°C, called the thermal comfort zone, understood as the zone in which the cow obtains, through normal thermoregulatory mechanisms, the adjustment of the internal temperature without any additional energy expenditure.

This second critical temperature point is ideal for milk production, since cattle have a greater capacity to withstand low temperatures than high ones.

In an observation that we carried out to find out the tolerance to heat of Holstein cows, in the shade and in bright sunlight, we were able to verify that the critical point of thermo-neutrality of cows kept in the shade was between 27-30 °C, with 60-70 % RH, while heat stress began to manifest between 29-32 °C, with 60-70 % RH.

This means that Cuban Holstein cows were tolerant to ambient heat, while they were kept in the shade of trees.

However, when exposed to the radiant action of the sun for one hour after 10 a.m., heat stress began to manifest at 25 °C, with 84 % RH.

A similar response was observed in a group of Cuban Siboney heifers exposed to radiant sun (Table 2-1). Although Cuban Siboney cows tolerated the combined action of high temperature and RH better when exposed to the sun, they also suffered from heat stress, since tolerance to environmental heat in the shade is not the same as tolerance to radiant sun, due to the additive heat effect caused by infrared radiation absorbed by the dark skin of this breed.

Table 2-1 Clinical indicator values of Siboney heifers exposed to sun

Stress Variables	RR 35-40 Weak	RR 41-70 Moderate	RR 71-75 Strong
Air temperature	24.5 ± 1.0	31.8 ± 3.5	33.5 ± 1.4
Relative humidity/%	87.9 ± 5.8	67.9 ± 10.6	64.8 ± 5.9
Respiratory Rate (RR)	a 36.0 ± 3.0	b $62,8 \pm 10$	c 73 ± 1.8
Rectal temperature	a 38.6 ± 0.5	b 39.5 ± 0.6	b 39.6 ± 0.2

Legend: a, b, c = different letters on the same line, significantly different $P < 0.05$.

These results allow us to understand that heat tolerance is an important quality for raising cattle in the tropics, but it does not make them invulnerable to environmental heat stress.

Nutritional stress

It is generally due to poor nutrition (quantitative or qualitative) received by cows during the livestock drought, which occurs during the dry season of the year.

Gradually, the daily ration does not satisfy the nutritional requirements of the animals, and they begin to use body reserves. Consequently, milk production is reduced, reproductive functions are suppressed and body mass decreases.

Although the ambient temperature is more moderate during this period, solar radiation is more intense and can also cause heat stress. The result is: effects on production, reproduction and health.

Water stress

Water stress occurs when the animal does not receive the water necessary to maintain the homeostasis of the organism. During livestock drought, pastures become lignified and dry, so the drinking water requirements increase.

An adult bovine must consume at least, 10 L/water/kg of DM ingested. It has been observed that a dairy cow can drink water every two hours, that is, twelve times a day and that the greatest water consumption occurs after the two main meals (dawn and dusk). It is estimated that a heifer needs about 90 L/day and a cow about 120.

It is important for the farmer to know the water requirements of grazing animals and to be concerned about ensuring their supply. Grazing animals must have the volumes of water they need at their disposal, otherwise, traveling long distances in search of it becomes an additional stressful agent.

The first clinical sign that indicates that the bovine animal is not ingesting enough water is the dryness of its feces. In more severe cases of dehydration, general weakness, dryness of the mucous membranes and muzzle, loss of skin elasticity and infrequent defecation, with blackish and dry feces, like horse droppings, occur.

How to prevent or mitigate the harmful effects of environmental stress and drought

From the above discussion it can be concluded that the most effective, economical and environmentally sustainable measure to prevent heat stress is to provide natural shade for animals by planting timber and fruit trees in pastures, in accordance with existing silvipastoral systems.

The reasons are numerous. Trees combine protection from the sun with the effect of decreasing radiation created by evaporated moisture from fresh leaves.

Shades arise as an alternative to protect animals from solar radiation and are considered the basic and most important modification of environmental conditions to decrease the effect of radiative heat.

They influence the rest of the components of the agricultural system by virtue of their shape and growth habits. Their leafy canopies influence the absorption of solar radiation, favor precipitation and air movement, while their extensive root systems fill large volumes of soil.

The soil substrate where they grow can also be altered by the absorption of water and nutrients, the redistribution of the latter as leaf litter, as well as the disturbing movement of roots and their possible associations with fungi and bacteria.

Trees can improve the productivity of an agro-ecosystem due to their influence on soil characteristics, microclimate, hydrology and other associated biological components.

Soil and its conservation

As is known, soil is the layer of organic and mineral materials that covers the earth's crust, in which plants develop their roots and take their food. The importance of soil in livestock farming was highlighted by the wise French zootechnician Andre Voisin (1964), when he wrote:

"The animal is the photograph of the soil".

Soil-climate interaction

Climate is an important soil-forming factor, as well as determining the type of vegetation that will develop naturally in each ecosystem.

In tropical climates, even more than in other climates, the natural vegetation that develops in each place constitutes a way of protecting the soil from the negative effects of the climate.

In the generality of soil degradation processes, both physical, chemical and biological, high radiation, intense rains and excessive heat contribute to accelerating these processes, together with wind, soil humidity and evapotranspiration.

The most important degradation processes are determined by the interaction of the climate with anthropic effects (caused by the action of man), for example, erosion, which affects almost all tropical territory, caused by deforestation and inadequate cultivation methods.

This erosion can be controlled and reduced when minimum tillage, contour sowing, strip cultivation, living barriers, terraces etc. are used, especially in mountainous or hilly areas.

In livestock farming, erosion can be controlled by avoiding overgrazing. The planting of trees and grasses constitutes a particularly effective plant cover in protecting the soil.

Chapter 3

Adjustment and evaluation of zootechnical actions

Contents:
Introduction. Selection of heifers for replacement. Importance of the pre-reproductive phase of females. Age and body mass at incorporation into reproduction. Reproductive management in breeding cattle. Evaluation of the reproductive performance of the herd. Interpretation of reproductive indices.

Introduction

Normal and regular reproduction is the essential basis for profitable cattle breeding, therefore, improving or selecting fertility and eliminating subfertility and sterility in cattle can mean a significant increase in milk or meat production.

From an economic point of view, definitive sterility is less important than low fertility, since completely sterile females are relatively few compared to the high number of females that suffer from some temporary disorder of their reproductive function. Therefore, it is necessary to know the factors capable of interfering in reproductive capacity, with the double objective of being able to maintain this fertility when it already exists and to restore it if it has decreased or disappeared.

Zootechnical actions

Selection of heifers for replacement

The adequate selection of replacement heifers is one of the essential aspects to achieve reproductive and productive improvement of any cattle herd.

Each dairy farm must have its own replacement by retaining, breeding and developing the daughters of its best cows, inseminated or ridden by the best bulls, according to the desired genotype.

To do this, it is necessary to record on an individual card the data required to carry out an acceptable qualitative evaluation of each animal, from birth until it reaches puberty.

The number of heifers to be selected will depend on the size of the herd. It is estimated that annually, about 20 % of the cows in production must be culled for different reasons. Thus, in a dairy farm of one hundred cows, 30 heifers must be prepared for replacement, of which the ten worst will be culled, in conformation, body mass at birth and age and body mass at puberty.

Importance of the pre-reproductive phase of females

This phase constitutes, in all females, the most important link in the chain of phenomena that lead to the beginning of sexual activity. Neglect of the animal during the period of growth and development, parasitism, and chronic malnutrition lead to delays in the onset of puberty, which is an important cause of the shortening of the reproductive life of female cattle.

It is known that for the heifer to reach puberty, it is necessary for it to reach ⅔ of the body mass it would have in its adult state and that the effect of body mass is even more important than age. Studies carried out on these aspects in different years, in livestock enterprises located in various provinces, provide interesting results that deserve to be discussed.

Age and body mass at incorporation into breeding

According to zootechnical standards, the incorporated heifer must be fit for reproduction, according to its age, weight and genital development. Body weight is more decisive than age.

Females with less than 300 kg of weight should not be incorporated into breeding, except in specific breeds. 100 % of heifers (conversion 18 months) should weigh 300 kg to be incorporated into breeding if they gain 500 g/day of live weight.

However, it is common to see how these principles are violated, and prepubescent and poorly developed animals are incorporated into breeding, with the belief that the reproductive process can be accelerated. Obviously, the inclusion of these unproductive animals in the herd constitutes an additional burden that causes economic losses to the dairy farm.

Being fit for reproduction means that the heifer that is incorporated into the reproductive program is pubescent and fertile, that is, it presents complete ovarian activity, with estrus, ovulation and formation of the corpus luteum.

To know this, it is necessary that each heifer be clinically diagnosed by a qualified technician. Only in this way can it be known if the heifers incorporated are truly in their reproductive phase. But the importance of this clinical examination lies not only in knowing if the heifer is sexually mature, but in checking if that female does not present any congenital disorder in its genital tract.

It is of no use for an animal to have an excellent genotype and external conformation, if its genital tract presents defect that limit or impede fertility or is a carrier of undesirable genes. For this reason, it is indicated to perform an external and internal clinical examination on each one of them.

The external examination must be directed to the inspection of the vulva, entrance to the vagina and the mammary gland. A small and narrow vulva, together with a poorly developed and inelastic udder, with rudimentary nipples of hard consistency, are present in cases of congenital ovarian hypoplasia and in Freemartins.

The persistence of the hymenal membrane together with the shortening or closure of the vaginal canal, but with a normal development of the udder, are concomitant symptoms of segmental aplasia of the Müllerian canals.

Rectal examination serves to corroborate the diagnosis but is not always necessary. The incidence of these three diseases is rare, but they must be considered to avoid the introduction of undesirable animals into the herd.

Reproductive management in breeding livestock

Extensive breeding

Despite the recognized benefits of AI, natural mating is still used in extensive breeding systems, in 85 % of cattle in Latin America and 95 % in Africa. Although extensive grazing is not the most suitable method for dairy or beef farming, it is necessary to include it in this work and dedicate a few paragraphs to its discussion, since, under the current conditions of livestock farming, it is materially impossible to do without this system of exploitation, which will continue for a long time.

The limiting factors are the low quality of the pastures, the rainfall regime and the poor quality of the soil. The short duration of the vegetative cycle of the pastures favors their maturation during the rainy season, to prevent drought from impeding their continued development in good conditions. Due to these limiting factors, female zebu cattle and their crosses adjust their reproductive cycle to the season of the year with the greatest and best availability of food, just as their African ancestors did.

Breeding livestock

Conceptually, it is the livestock farm whose main purpose is the development of the offspring to produce meat (without milking) in various forms of organization of the management of the herds and reproduction techniques, generally natural mating.

For this type of extensive breeding, animals of the zebu genotype are used that, due to their rusticity and natural resistance, can survive the unfavorable conditions of the tropical climate, with a minimum of attention from man. Generally, it is in remote places, difficult to access, with poor soils, natural pastures and high infestation of bushes and undergrowth.

The unfavorable characteristics of the herds of zebu cattle for breeding are age at first birth of 3-4 years, interpartal intervals of 500 days or more, birth rates of 30-50 %, perinatal losses of more than 20 %, low proportion and quality of female replacements, lack of systematization of weaning.

The factors that influence poor reproductive performance are inherent to the particularities of Zebu cattle, which are usually early born, with ovarian activity that is inhibited by lactation and the suckling of the calf.

The cause of lactation anestrus is that the suckling of the calf, in addition to stimulating the release of oxytocin by the posterior pituitary gland for the "letdown" of milk and prolactin by the anterior pituitary gland, induces the secretion of endorphins in the CNS, which inhibit the release of GnRH, all of which leads to anestrus.

As the calf grows, it begins to ingest other foods apart from milk and no longer suckles as frequently.

The decrease in the frequency of breastfeeding causes less endorphins to be released and the inhibition they exerted on the hypothalamus gradually ceases and GnRH is released in increasingly wider and more frequent pulses, with the subsequent release of FSH and LH, which travel to the ovary and stimulate the complete process of folliculogenesis.

As the suckling of the calf is not the only factor involved in lactation anestrus, sometimes the resumption of ovarian activity does not occur until weaning or even after.

The long periods of anestrus are increased by the loss of body mass caused by malnutrition suffered during the period of livestock drought.

It can be said that the reproductive efficiency of extensive breeding depends on the exploitation factors that I list below and on which work must be done to maintain them:

1) Suitability of the breeding bulls used.
2) Aptitude of cows and heifers.
3) Herd organization and control.
4) Adequate reproductive management techniques.

Reproductive management variants

The reproductive management variants in breeding cattle include artificial insemination, directed mating, natural mating, the creation of patios and gestation farms.

Artificial insemination

This is the biotechnology that guarantees the greatest responses to selection and has, among other advantages, the possibility of accurately recognizing the paternity of the offspring and achieving higher fertility and birth rates.

Directed mating

This is natural mating but directed by man. It offers similar advantages to AI, with the disadvantage that it requires numerous bulls of high genetic value that must be cared for and maintained. In Cuba it is used in small herds of private breeders.

Natural mating

Mating occurs without human intervention. This is the form of reproduction used in extensive breeding.

Courtyards

These are reproductive management variants, where a group of females live with bulls to facilitate their mating in a natural way. Depending on the number of animals, two types are recognized.

Single yard

It is made up of 20-25 females and a breeding bull. This management variant allows the fertility of the parents to be controlled individually and the paternity of the offspring to be determined.

Multiple yard

the number of females can reach 200, to be served by a group of 8 to 10 bulls. That is, maintaining a ratio of one bull for 20 or 25 cows. With this variant, paternity control is not possible.

To improve the reproductive performance of the animals kept in the aforementioned yards, two reproductive management methods have been used that have been shown to increase the birth rate. These are: the gestation farm and the breeding season.

Gestation farm

It consists of a natural pasture, 81 to 94 ha, that allows maximum loads of 200 animals. This farm must have a perimeter fence in good condition, with radial grazing and be subdivided into 6 to 8 paddocks and a central corral. In addition, it must have a trap to secure the animals during the clinical-gynecological examination, a work corral, water troughs, feeders and saltshakers.

This farm not only functions as a temporary site that favors couplings, but is also an option for raising developing females, which will replace the less productive cows the following year.

The basis of the diet is natural pastures and as forage it is recommended to sow areas of King grass, Cuba CT-115 and sugar cane of forage varieties. Protein banks should be established with Leucaena or other regionalized legumes and silvipastoral systems, if the soil and climate conditions allow it.

The supply of mineral formulations and common salt is important. The supply of multi-nutritional blocks can be an excellent option to supplement the calories and minerals necessary for reproduction.

The objectives pursued with the establishment of these farms are to increase calf births to 70 % or more, facilitate the development of yearlings so that they can serve as replacements in the coming mating season and rid the herds of females unfit for reproduction.

Complementary technical actions

Reproductive management includes previous actions by the veterinarian-zootechnician that include the external and internal clinical examination of females and males, to discard defective animals or those in poor physical condition, before entering the farm. The cows that are incorporated must be weaned and the heifers must have the required body development.

If natural mating is used, it is essential that all bulls be measured and verified for their ability to mount the female in heat. Due to its importance, I include in this part, little-known aspects about the sexual behavior of zebu bulls in extensive breeding.

Sexual behavior of Zebu bulls in natural mating

In general, Zebu bulls are more phlegmatic and react more slowly to a female in heat than *Bos taurus* bulls, but slow response should not be confused with sexual apathy that manifests itself in semi-frigidity or constitutional frigidity that has a hereditary origin. A reaction time test of seven Zebu bulls, faced with Zebu cows in spontaneous heat, showed that all of them performed the first service within 15 minutes of the start of the test and some even gave up to two services. A reaction time of 18,4 ± 9,0 minutes was also observed in Zebu bulls under the artificial vagina collection regime.

When a Zebu bull is introduced into a herd of cows, he faces several obstacles that he must overcome in order to be able to service these females. First, he must establish his dominance over the dominant cows. An active cow may compete for the attention of the male.

An active cow may compete for the bull's attention by butting him on the flank, but the bull will often mount other females in heat as well.

When a group of 5 to 6 bulls is introduced into a herd, a struggle to establish the social hierarchy takes place among them. The bull that wins dominance is the one that will do most of the mounting.

Subordinate bulls only have the opportunity to participate when the dominant male reduces his sexual activity. If the bulls used in the yards are not selected for their ability to move and mount, good birth results cannot be expected. However, in practice, this issue is not given the attention it deserves. In very few cases, the breeding bulls are checked for their mounting ability, nor are they subjected to external and internal andrological examinations.

In herds where new heifers are introduced, it is necessary to include young bulls (24 to 36 months old), which are more active and more interested in them than older dominant bulls. In addition, physical compatibility must be taken into account when mating.

Older, very corpulent bulls find it more difficult to mount less corpulent heifers. Some heifers may not withstand the jumping and hugging of very heavy bulls.

Measuring the ability to mount

The sexual behavior of the male is determined by his anatomical and functional integrity and by his genetic constitution, expressed in the speed of response and interest in stimuli emanating from the female in heat. The speed of reaction and the intensity of expression of the primary sexual reflexes are essential components of sexual libido.

In practice, the sexual behavior of the male is measured by the reaction time, which is the time between the ejaculatory prelude and ejaculation. The evaluation is based on the speed with which a bull performs courtship, erection of the penis, jumping, hugging, searching, introduction, ejaculation and dismounting.

To evaluate a bull's sexual libido and his ability to mount, it is necessary to confront him with a female in heat, whether natural or induced, and observe his performance. The service capacity is a measure of the number of services achieved by a bull, under a given time and conditions.

This test must be done by confronting several females in heat with a given number of bulls (6 females: 4 bulls) for a period of 30 minutes.

When examining the male in action, it must be taken into account that virility depends more on the speed of the act than on the intensity of the excitement; thus, some bulls try to make the jump before the erection begins; in others, the erection is incomplete and the penetration of the penis is compromised. Conversely, the male can remain restless around the female and yet not attempt the jump at any time. In such cases, it is necessary to assess whether the problem is due to the animal itself or to extrinsic factors, such as the presence of strangers during the test. The possible presence of erectile disorders due to the shortening of the penile S and the persistence of the preputial frenulum should also be taken into account.

Mating season

This is a reproductive management variant, applicable to any form of herd organization, consisting of promoting the mating of animals, bringing them together for a period of 3 or 4 months, at the beginning of the months of greatest availability of pastures.

The advantages offered by the mating season are that it increases birth rates, and concentrates births and weaning's to avoid calf losses, in addition to facilitating the work of the breeder.

On the other hand, mating, selection, pregnancy diagnosis, birth, weaning, identification, weighing, deworming, vaccination, veterinary investigations and pasture management programs can be better planned.

Each farmer must determine the most convenient months for its establishment, adjusting to the type of microclimate of the farm or ranch in each region. In the case of Cuba, the most propitious months to establish the breeding season in Cuba are from June to September or from June to October, depending on the beginning of the rainiest season of the year.

Temporary weaning

To minimize the effect of calf suckling on the duration of postpartum anestrus in Zebu cows, a management procedure has been tested, consisting of separating the calf from its mother every 18 days, to prevent it from suckling for three consecutive days.

This form of restricted suckling has been called temporary weaning 18x3. The results obtained ranged between 0% and 27 % of heat in three groups of animals observed.

Due to the poor results achieved and the laborious handling, especially with the separation and feeding of the calf for three days, in addition to the mother-child stress that it causes, this management variant has little chance of being accepted and generalized in livestock practice.

Evaluation of the reproductive performance of the herd

Reproductive indices

Reproductive indices allow us to identify areas for improvement, set realistic reproductive goals, monitor progress, and identify problems at an early stage. They can also be used to uncover historical management problems in the herd.

Reproductive management of a herd must be a joint task between the farmer and the veterinary zootechnician, since the main objective is to optimize reproductive results.

Most indices for a herd are calculated as the average of individual performance. In small herds, the evaluation of reproductive performance can go from the average of the herd to the individual performance of the cow.

Reproductive status of the herd

The first assessment that must be made is related to the reproductive status of the herd, since this assessment measures the effectiveness of the actions developed in feeding, reproductive management, and veterinary care.

The reproductive status of an ideal herd of one hundred cows, shown below, can serve as a comparative pattern to evaluate any other.

Table 3-1 Ideal reproductive status of the herd

Reproductive Status	Desirable value(%)
Cows with lactations < 60 days	10 - 12
Inseminated or mated	25 - 30
Confirmed pregnancy	> 50
Opens < 120 days	≤ 5
Recent delivery	≤ 10

The group of inseminated or mated cows that have not yet been diagnosed as pregnant is the one with the greatest source of variation due to the variability in herd fertility and the time at which pregnancy diagnosis is made.

The proportion could decrease by almost half when pregnancy diagnosis is made early (35-50 days). On the other hand, the frequency of monthly calvings should be 7 to 8, which is equivalent to a birth rate of 84-90 %.

Record control

It is obvious that, to process and evaluate the reproductive data of the herd, it is necessary to ensure that the dairy farm has good control of the reproductive performance of each female and that all data is recorded punctually and correctly on the control card, which must be kept by the inseminating technician.

This reproductive control card contains the necessary data to know the historical background of the animal, from the time it is incorporated into the reproduction program, to each of the births it has had. The most recent events are also recorded, such as: date of the last birth, date of inseminations after each birth, date of gestation, etc.

A dairy farm, ranch or livestock company that does not have records of productive and reproductive data of its animals, from birth, will not be able to aspire to improve its livestock, since the selection criteria can only be obtained from the measurement and recording of that data, in a lasting manner.

Obtaining and calculating

It should be noted that no reproductive index alone allows a definitive conclusion to be reached about what is happening in the herd, so it is necessary to obtain and evaluate them as a whole and interpret their interrelations.

Reproductive indices can be calculated manually using a digital calculator from the primary data obtained from each individual card. Although manual calculation is laborious and cumbersome, especially when the herd is larger than 50 animals, it is a feasible option to use. It is best to do it between two people, one looking for the data on the card and the other writing down the data in a model created for this purpose.

If it is a matter of evaluating the reproductive data of a farm or livestock company, it is best to use computerized programs or applications, recognized for their simplicity and effectiveness.

If you do not have these programs, you can use the Microsoft Excel spreadsheet, in the versions of the Microsoft Office operating system.

This application provides communication facilities to the user, as it includes a general help system and does not require extensive programming knowledge.

In addition, it facilitates the performance of mathematical operations through formulas and numbers stored in "electronic cells" that can be used again and again to analyze the sensitivity of the input data.

Interpretation of reproductive indices

Interval calving first insemination ICFI)

This is the time, in days, between birth and the first insemination. It often coincides with the first postpartum estrus and is generally recorded on the reproduction control cards.

Its analysis allows us to infer how females are responding reproductively under the feeding and management conditions to which they are subjected (postpartum anestrus) and gives an early idea of the duration of the birth-gestation interval.

Uterine involution and its relationship with the first postpartum estrus

The duration of uterine involution depends on many conditions: quality of feed, milk production, age, birth process, puerperium, etc. It has been confirmed that, in general, puerperal uterine involution varies between 30 and 50 days and is almost complete at the time of the first estrus. The incorporation of the cow into a new reproductive cycle depends on the resumption of the estrous cycle, which generally begins with the appearance of the first postpartum heat.

It has been proven that the first postpartum heat in dairy cows occurs between 4 and 6 weeks on average and in beef producers between 4 and 7 weeks or more.

However, in well-fed dairy cows the first heat can appear as early as 7-15 days postpartum, when uterine involution has not yet been completed. This means that the cow should not be inseminated or mounted before 50 days.

This period during which uterine involution occurs is called, in livestock jargon, *recentinage* and the cow in this state is the *recentina*.

Thus, in livestock practice, recentinage is used as a reproductive category. The remaining reproductive categories are inseminated, pregnant and empty cows.

The voluntary waiting period and the ICFI

The voluntary waiting period is the period, in days, that the man decides must be waited for the cow to be inseminated or mounted after calving. This waiting period can coincide with or go beyond the completion of uterine involution, which normally occurs between 45-50 days.

The voluntary waiting period is quite short, if one considers that the female reaches her highest fertility potential after 60-70 days postpartum.

If the cow is inseminated at 60 days postpartum, she goes into the inseminated category. If that inseminated cow does not return to service, or in other words, does not show heat again, it is assumed that she is pregnant, but she does not go into the pregnant category until pregnancy is confirmed. This is done by means of rectal examination, three months after insemination or mating.

Once pregnancy is confirmed, the cow is then placed in the pregnant category and is marked as such to differentiate it from the rest. If after 50 days the cow does not show heat (anestrus), it is then placed in the empty cow category. The empty cow category depends on the duration of the period considered as physiological sexual rest after delivery, in a certain genotype and the availability of food available to supply the herd.

Nutritional and management factors influencing the duration of the ICFI

The reappearance of the estrous cycle after delivery depends on internal and external factors which can act individually or in combination.

High milk production contributes to increasing the ICFI duration. Cows during their maximum production suffer from an energy imbalance as they cannot access the necessary nutrients that the feed provides and must take them from organic reserves. This causes a decrease in their body mass. During lactation, the secretion of PIF decreases, as does that of LH-RH, with the consequent restriction of pituitary gonadotropins, thus affecting follicular maturation and ovulation.

As regards the milking system, it has been observed that cows subjected to a regime of 4 milkings per day have an average *interval-calving-first-estrus* (ICFE) of 69 days, while those milked twice come into heat at around 46 days. Cows that suckle their calves can reach average ICFE of 72 days. This is related to the mechanism of regulation of lactation and sexual functions already mentioned.

The presence of the calf with its mother also influences the maintenance of milk production. Separation from the calf or its early death changes the complex neuro-hormonal lactogenic control system, resulting in a rapid onset of sexual activity. This is observed in some beef breeds, and especially in Zebu, which, when nursing their calves, show a delay in the first postpartum heat, which considerably lengthens the ICFE.

The postpartum feeding level also closely matches the duration of the ICFE. Dairy cows with a high feeding level come into heat earlier than those with a poor nutritional level. The decisive factor for the resumption of the oestrus cycle after calving is the maintenance of a constant body mass of the mothers.

There is a close relationship between the ICFE and the ICFI, since in practice it is the ICFI that is recorded on the cards, especially when the voluntary waiting period is over.

ICFI analysis allows us to know how females are responding reproductively to the exploitation and management conditions to which they are subjected and gives us an advance idea of the duration of the birth-gestation interval.

Physiological postpartum anestrus period

This is the absence of estrus from the time the cow calves until the current date. It is obtained by counting the days from the date of the last calving to the current day. The figure obtained in this way indicates the actual time that the animal has not shown sexual activity and serves to assess the individual and collective situation of the herd in the face of agro-ecological, exploitation and management conditions and to take the appropriate measures to shorten it.

If the prevailing environmental conditions are unfavorable or there are problems with food availability or poor management, it is to be expected that the return to sexuality will be delayed and postpartum anestrus will occur, prolonged. The duration of the physiological postpartum rest therefore depends on the conditions.

By determining the ICFI and organizing it in a frequency distribution, the duration of recent past anestrus and its incidence can be known retrospectively. Except for Zebu breeds, in well-fed cows of any genotype, anestrus lasting less than 60 days can be considered physiological. In cows receiving an average level of nutrition, anestrus lasting up to 90 days is common. Postpartum anestrus lasting more than 90 days indicates the existence of a negative energy balance in the female, which prevents the resumption of ovarian activity.

Interval calving conception (ICC)

This is the time between the last calving and the fertilizing insemination or mating. This index is also known as the period of services or open days, but these names can be confusing for non-experts. The ICC is one of the indexes with the most predictable value, since it includes the duration of the ICFI, plus the days that the females needed to be fertilized;

that is, it measures the degree of fertility that the female had before the inseminations carried out.

A short ICFI, with a long ICC, indicates that service repetitions have occurred, while a long ICFI, with an ICC equal to or slightly greater than the ICFI, indicates that anestrus has occurred.

The duration of the ICC should not be calculated from the number of services per conception, since the intervals between inseminations are generally longer than the duration of the normal sexual cycle (18-21 days).

Calving interval (CI)

This is the time between two consecutive births and is used to measure a cow's ability to produce a live calf in the shortest possible time.

Ideally, a farmer should have a CI of as short as 365 days for his cows, which is equivalent to producing one calf per year. But for this to happen, the ICC should not exceed 90 days.

It is interesting to know that this excellent reproductive response could only be achieved in five of the 10 herds of pure *Bos taurus* cows (50 %) and in five of the 20 crossbred herds that we studied.

Long interpartum intervals represent great economic losses if they are left unattended, not only in intensive livestock farming, but also in the conditions of moderately intensive and extensive farming, where work must be done to improve the environmental conditions that limit reproduction and livestock production.

Services per conception (SC) or conception rate (CR)

It is also known as the insemination index or coital index. It expresses the number of services necessary to obtain a recognized pregnancy. The term "services" refers to the heat itself, regardless of the number of inseminations or mounts performed in that heat; that is, if a cow is inseminated or mounted two or three times in the same heat and because of those inseminations becomes pregnant, the number of SC of that cow is 1, since it is counted as a single service.

To calculate it, all the services received by the females are added up, in the period of one year and divided by the number that became pregnant. Please note that heifers should not be mixed with cows.

In general, heifers have a higher fertility potential than cows and therefore SCs reach an average value of 1 to 1.2. If a high percentage of heifers require more than two services per conception, one should suspect poor quality of the semen used or problems with the application of the A.I. technique. In *Bos taurus* cows inseminated in Cuba, averages of 1.6 to 2.7 services/conception are reported and 1.3 to 1.8 in Zebu and their crosses.

Conception rate at first insemination

This index also measures the fertility potential of the bull, but, above all, the technical efficiency of the inseminator, who is the one who applies the biotechnology. For this reason, it is important to know the range of normal fertility potential of the different genotypes in the country.

To calculate this figure, all females that were pregnant at the first service or mounted for the first time after delivery are added up, multiplied by one hundred and divided by the total number of females inseminated for the first time.

A percentage of pregnancies at the first service of more than 70 % is considered excellent, 70 % as good, 60-51 % as acceptable and less than 50 % as poor.

Insemination technicians can achieve good technical efficiency if they take into account important aspects such as: not performing a single service, inseminating at appropriate times, using a suspicious bull to determine whether the female is in the receptive phase of heat, not inseminating females that are not really in heat, respecting the voluntary waiting period, depositing the semen inside the cervical canal, not using semen in poor condition, among others.

Total pregnancy rate

It measures the percentage of females diagnosed as pregnant, of the total herd. It is obtained by dividing the number of pregnant females, by the total number of females examined. The result is multiplied by one hundred. This indicator has a limited utilitarian value.

Birth rate

This percentage is the one that best measures the reproductive performance of the herd, because it reveals the result of all the factors that affect the reproductive performance of the herd.

There are two ways to calculate it depending on whether heifers are included or not.

$$\text{Birth rate} = \frac{\text{N. of calves born alive} \times 100}{\text{Average number of cows on farm}}$$

$$\text{Birth rate} = \frac{\text{N. of calves born alive} \times 100}{\text{N. of cows + 50\% of heifers over 18 months old}}$$

For the conditions of Cuban livestock farming, it is preferable to use the first form, since the age of incorporation of heifers into reproduction varies greatly, in the different genotypes and livestock companies.

For dairy cattle, a birth rate of 80 % is excellent, 70% or more is good, more than 60 % is acceptable and less than 50 % is bad.

For Zebu cattle, in conditions of extensive breeding and free mounting, a birth rate of 70 % is excellent, 64 % is good and less than 50 % is bad.

Non births rate

This is given by the percentage of females considered pregnant that should have given birth and do not do so due to: abortions, diagnostic errors and deaths. It should not be higher than 3-5 %. When this percentage exceeds 5 %, possible conflicts of interest should be suspected in the technical staff who receive a better salary when they report more females as pregnant. Professionals must be alert to the commission of fraud in records, especially when many abortions and diagnostic errors are reported.

Chapter 4

Proposal for an agroforestry project

Content:
Introduction. Project outline. Multipurpose tree planting, a solution to sustainable livestock development. Additional activities for project implementation. Task breakdown. Improvement of the livestock agroecosystem. Expected results.

Introduction

This chapter is aimed at entrepreneurs who own farms or livestock farms and are interested in improving the ecosystem where their animals are raised.

What we propose is not a finished project but rather an outline that can be adapted to any animal exploitation system, mainly where the soils are poor and devoid of trees, regardless of the size of the farm or farm.

Before executing the project, a feasibility analysis and a cost calculation for the necessary inputs are required.

In my experience, seedlings are the most difficult materials to obtain, due to their variety, quantity and prices.

Therefore, to minimize costs, I recommend purchasing the seeds and planting them in nylon bags with a cubic liter capacity, or any similar container and creating your own nurseries, as explained in the description of the variants.

It is essential to carry out an inspection of the local and regional environment and to investigate the existence of timber and fruit trees that best adapt to the topographic characteristics of your farm. Select those species that grow faster, are resistant to drought and have good foliage.

Project outline

Topic

Multipurpose arborization, a solution to sustainable livestock development

Justification

In most tropical countries, natural shade areas on farms or livestock farms are extremely scarce, so animals are subjected to moderate to strong heat stress, which results in effects on fertility, milk and meat production.

In addition, the lack of trees affects the rainfall regime with the consequent shortage of pastures and the impoverishment of soil quality. On the other hand, numerous hectares of land not suitable for grazing remain uncultivated.

All these factors make the productivity of livestock systems in the tropics low and economically unprofitable.

General objective

The objective of this project is to apply arborization and reforestation in cattle, goat and sheep farms, with a more biological concept, in accordance with the shade requirements for animals, pastures and soils, supported by integrity and biodiversity, in accordance with the principles of sustainable agriculture.

By improving the agroecosystem where animals are raised, we hope to achieve an increase in milk and meat production, with better reproductive efficiency.

Another important objective is to contribute to reducing the cost of milk and meat production, from additional production of wood, firewood, fruits, honey and their by-products, which could make animal husbandry more profitable.

Materials and methods to be used

It should be noted that not all farms are suitable for use in the agrosilvipastoral system due to the costs involved and the natural differences that make up the microclimates.

It is therefore necessary, over time, to determine and define the most suitable areas for each component, considering factors such as soil quality, topography, previous use, ease of access and others that are considered important for the success of the project.

Therefore, a characterization of each of the dairy farms or farms will be made with respect to soil, topography and population of existing trees, to know what the requirements are for tree planting and the species that should be planted and ensure their survival.

The tree planting of each dairy farm will be done on the borders, marginal areas and within the grazing areas.

The species planted on the borders must be regionalized to ensure their viability and productivity. The distance between the seedlings will be 2-3 meters, depending on the species. An attempt will be made to intersperse timber and fruit tree species.

Timber and fruit trees will be planted in marginal areas. The planting distance for timber species will be 2-3 meters and for fruit trees 4-6 meters depending on their leafiness.

The tree species to be planted in the grazing areas are those described in Chapter 2. This selection considered the leafiness required for animal shade, combined with that necessary for the development of pastures.

The number of seedlings to be planted will be 25 to 100/ha, depending on the existing population and the species to be planted in each ha.

Since in livestock farming the arborization of grazing areas is the most difficult problem to solve due to the predatory effect of the animal on the plants, eight variants are proposed that provide alternatives for the fulfillment of this task.

The materials required for the project are shovels, picks, a hoe, an auger for making holes in the ground, attached to a tractor, organic fertilizer or humus from bovine manure, and seeds from wood and fruit trees that are selected in the project design. The seeds will be used to be sown in nurseries to obtain seedlings that will be transferred to nylon bags with a cubic liter capacity, until they reach the height and foliage most suitable for their final transplant.

The hole must be the same depth as the roots and a diameter of at least *three times their size*. This allows for rapid root growth and offers greater stability to the seedling.

Before placing the seedling in the hole, any wrapping or packing material that may be around the roots must be removed.

After placing the plant in the center of the hole, the hole will be filled with loose soil, making sure that the roots are well covered and that there are no air pockets. Compacting the soil around the tree should be avoided, as this will hinder root growth.

Each newly planted seedling should be watered adequately to settle the soil and provide the plant with the moisture necessary for its initial growth.

In addition, apply a layer of mulch around the tree to help retain moisture and control undesirable weeds.

Variant 1

For areas invaded by marabou or other undesirable species that are part of the net productive area of the farm or ranch.

Species to be planted:

Eucalyptus globulus, *Swietenia macrophylla* (Honduran mahogany), *Swieteria Khaya* (African mahogany), Neem, *Pines* (Pine) and others.

Planting distance in meters: 2x2 and 2x2,5.

This high density of 2,000 to 2,500 plants per hectare is part of the control plan for undesirable invasive plants such as marabou.

Characteristics of the location: Varied.

Management:

Thinning to allow the establishment or appearance of grass spontaneously. After the plantation has been established and the undesirable plants have been controlled, as many thinning's will be carried out as required by the area.

Objective:

Obtaining wood, seeds, medicinal preparations, cujes, honey.

Variant 2

Areas with young or maternity cattle

Unpalatable species will be planted; for cattle that cause minimum animal damage during the first 2-3 years.

Species to plant:

Neem and pine.

Planting distance in meters: From 5x10 to 10x20.

Characteristics of the location:

Flat or undulating.

Management:

During the first two years only cultural attention and later pruning or thinning according to the needs.

Objective:

Shade for pastures and animals, seeds and wood.

Variant 3

Rotation of forage areas with considerable loss of soil fertility for areas of various crops and later to produce pasture seeds.

Species to plant:

Fruit trees, Neem, Eucalyptus, Leucaena, wood, Pigeon pea.

Planting distance in meters: From 5x10 to 10x20.

Characteristics of the location:

Flat or undulating topography with good to medium fertility.

Management:

During the first two years only cultural attention and later pruning or thinning according to the needs.

Objective:

Support of fences, production of forage (browsing), new posts, shade, firewood, honey.

Variant 4

Borders

It consists of planting a row or line of trees along the entire border, road, roads, accesses, simultaneously with the living fences.

Species to plant: fruit trees, especially coconut and some timber trees according to soil conditions.

Planting distance in meters: 5x10.

Characteristics of the location: Variable.

Management: cultural activities and thinning according to requirements.

Living fences

Species that reproduce by cuttings: *Erythrina berteroana, Echinodorus grisebachii* (Amazon sword plant), *E. poeppigiana, Gliricidia sepium* (quickstick), *Jatropha curcas* (Purging nut). *Bursera simaruba* (Gumbo-limbo) *Spondias sp* (Hog plums) or other similar trees. Interplant with fruit trees.

Planting distance in meters: 2 to 3.

Management: Pruning at the end of flowering and to produce new propagules.

Objective: Support of fences, production of forage (browsing), new posts, shade, firewood, honey.

Variant 5

Corners

It is indicated for fenced grazing areas in small plots. It is planted diagonally to protect them from damage caused by animals while grazing.

Species to plant:

Eucalyptus, Neem, fruit trees, etc. One plant per corner.

Planting distance in meters:

One meter from the mother or corner.

Characteristics of the location:

Variable. Use of unused corners.

Management:

Cultural care.

Objective:

Taking advantage of inaccessible areas.

Variant 6

Oasis

It consists of the establishment of groups of trees (25-100) of varied geometric shapes.

These oases will be located mainly in the corners; but they can be located in other parts of the area, taking advantage of peaks or hills that could be rocky with very low production of grass, waterholes, etc.

Species to plant: Eucalyptus, Neem, hardwood species and fruit trees.

Planting distance in meters: 3x3.

Characteristics of the location:

Hard-to-reach areas. Sloping, rocky areas.

Management:

Agro-technical attention, thinning, some pruning.

Objective:

Take advantage of non-cultivable or grazing areas.

Additional activities for project implementation

Discussions will be provided to the dairy farm staff to create a culture aimed at the care and preservation of trees as a way to increase livestock production.

In each dairy farm, small nurseries will be built, especially for fruit trees, to produce the seedlings necessary for their area. The organic fertilizer required for the germination and growth of the seedlings will be obtained from the cowsheds' manure, processed in the form of humus or from any other source.

These nurseries would be attended by the cowboys themselves as part of their integral dairy work content.

In the area of the farm or ranch, one or more nurseries will be built attended by personnel assigned to this task. These nurseries would ensure the seedlings that are most difficult to acquire.

The number of seedlings to be produced will be determined by the characterization made of the forest population of the dairy farms.

If the population to be forested is 25 to 100 seedlings per hectare, the total hectare of the farm or ranch must be added up and the tree planting of 10 % of the area or 20 % at most must be calculated.

Care will be taken to ensure the survival of the seedlings, the development of the plants, the beginning of fruit production, the degree of leafiness and the benefits provided to the pastures.

In parallel with the planting of trees, efforts will be made to create the necessary conditions for improving pastures, creating areas planted with legumes to provide a satisfactory level of protein, forage areas, building silos, haylofts, etc. to ensure good nutrition for animals throughout the year.

Task breakdown

Improving the livestock agroecosystem

The planting of trees will include the slopes of the embankment that gives access to the dairy farms, planting fruit trees on both sides, 3-4 meters apart along lanes.

The methods and procedures to follow when planting borders, marginal areas and pastures have been described in general materials and methods.

The size of the areas to be planted with trees and the planting distances will determine the total number of seedlings needed. The most desirable thing is to try to plant trees on at least 20 % of the area per year.

To carry out the work with quality and precision, it is advisable to appoint a brigade or team of five or six men, dedicated especially to this task. They would oversee organizing, carrying out the daily work, acquiring the seeds of timber and fruit trees indicated in the project and creating and maintaining the nurseries to obtain the necessary seedlings.

Keep in mind that a project of this magnitude requires the collaboration of many people, that is, community members, family, friends, children from primary schools (obtaining fruit seeds and school nurseries).

Expected results

With the improvement of the agroecosystem, in the medium term (5-7 years) it is possible to create a thermal environment more favorable for milk production, which allows increases of 5 to 10 % per lactation period and an increase in the fertility rate of 5 to 10 % in the hottest season of the year.

Ensuring that animals have an adequate nutritional plan throughout the year will reduce morbidity and mortality in livestock, with the consequent increase in economic benefits.

Facilitating the occurrence of rainfall and therefore a better availability of moisture to the soil to satisfy, to a greater extent, the water demand of pastures and trees.

Naturally protecting soils against water erosion and raising the levels of organic matter, so that soils improve qualitatively.

The availability of greater quantities of wood, firewood, fruits and honey would constitute a considerable additional economic contribution.

At the end of the project, the farms will have a forest potential of thousands of cubic meters of wood and firewood. Each honey tree could produce one kg of honey per year.

Each apiary of 25 hives produces honey, wax, propolis and pollen worth several hundred dollars. Each fruit tree can produce 15-20 kg of fruit per year, which is an additional profit.

This set of benefits can result in a substantial reduction in the cost of milk and meat production. In addition, it will favor environmental conservation, contribute to improving the community's standard of living, reduce the destructive effects of storms and improve the beauty of the rural landscape and therefore the mental state of the local population.

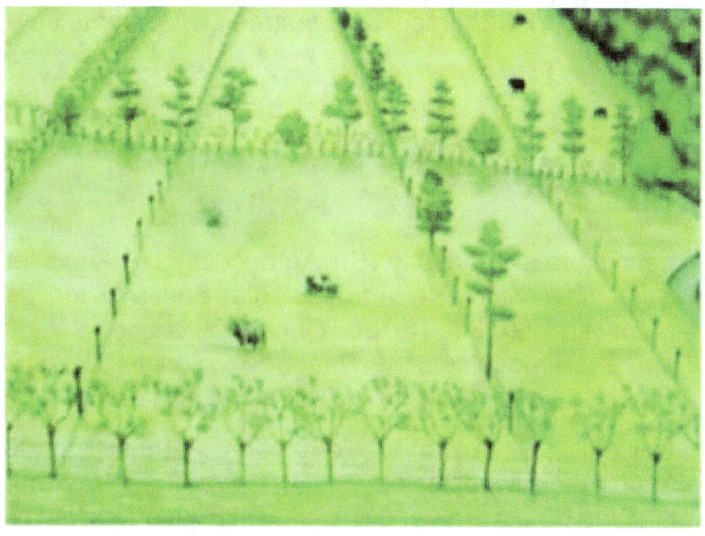

Bibliography

Alba, L. O., Koutinhouin, B.: 1995. La disfunción del cuerpo lúteo asociada a algunos factores climáticos en el síndrome repetición de servicios, en vacas Holstein de Cuba. VI Congreso Nacional de C. Veterinarias, La Habana.

Alba, L. O., Koutinhouin, B., Torres, L.: 1995. Estimación del efecto del estrés de calor ambiental, utilizando el índice de calor sofocante (ICS) y su relación con la tasa de fertilidad de las vacas Holstein. VI Congreso Nacional de C. Veterinarias, La Habana.

Alba, L. O., Koutinhouin, B., Torres, L.:1995. Efecto del estrés calor natural, sobre la respuesta ovárica y la capacidad fertilizadora de los gametos, en vacas Holstein. VI Congreso Nacional de C. Veterinarias, La Habana.

Altieri, M.: 1992. El rol ecológico de la biodiversidad en agro-sistemas. Agroecología y desarrollo. U. C. Berkeley-CLADES.

Altieri, M.: 1997. Bases agroecológicas para una agricultura sustentable. En Agroecología y Agricultura Sostenible. Módulo 1 Agroecología: Bases históricas y teóricas. 122-133. 1ra Ed. Consorcio Latinoamericano sobre Agroecología y Desarrollo Social. CLADES-Programa de Educación a Distancia, La Habana.

Calzadilla, E., Leyva, R., Torres, J. y Martínez A.: 1997. Sistemas silvipastoriles en la Sierra Maestra, Cuba: Árboles de sombra en pastizales. III Encuentro Nacional de Agricultura Orgánica, Universidad Central, L.V. Cuba.

FAO-1993.: La diversidad en la naturaleza un patrimonio valioso. Dirección de Información, FAO, Roma.

Farrel, J.: 1997. Sistemas agroforestales, en Agroecología y Agricultura sostenible. Módulo 2. Diseño y manejo de sistemas agrícolas sostenibles. 1ra Ed. Consorcio Latinoamericano sobre Agroecología y Desarrollo Social. CLADES-Programa de Educación a Distancia, La Habana.

Galvez G., Jordán, H., Crespo G., Castillo E., Cino D., Febles G. García R., Trujillo G., Molina A., Reyes, J., Senra A., Febles J., Cuesta A., Alonso C., Durán J. y Fernández L. 1996. Estudio de sistemas de pastoreo y su influencia en la relación suelo-planta-animal. II Simposio sobre agricultura sostenible. X Seminario Científico del INCA, La Habana.

García R.: 1995. La conversión hacia una agricultura orgánica. Agricultura Orgánica (1):8-14.

Gómez María Elena, Rodríguez Lylian, Murgertio E., Rios Clara Inés, Heman C., Hemando C., Molina E., Molina J.: 1995. Árboles y Arbustos Forrajeros Utilizados en la Alimentación Animal como Fuente Proteica: Matarratón (Gliricidia sepium), Nacedero (Trichanthera gigantea) y Botón de Oro Tithonia diversifolia). Ed. Centro para la investigación en Sistemas Sostenibles de Producción Agropecuaria. Fundación CIPAV, Cali.

Ingraham, R., Guillete D. & Wagner, W.: 1974. Relationship of temperature and humidity to conception rate of Holstein cow in subtropical climate. J. Dairy Sci. 58(88):71-76.

Lecha, L.: 1979. Las condiciones de calor sofocante en la región Central de Cuba. Instituto de Meteorología, Academia de Ciencias de Cuba, Santa Clara.

Lecha, L. y Chugaev, A.:1989. La bioclimatología y algunas de sus aplicaciones en condiciones de clima tropical húmedo. Editorial Academia, La Habana, 1-35.

Machuca, L. A.: 1987. Presentación del estrés de calor en hembras ¾ Holstein x ¼ cebú en el clima tropical húmedo con vertientes interiores secas de Guantánamo. Tesis de doctorado. Departamento de Ciencias Biológicas. Universidad de Oriente, Cuba.

Morais, M. y Espinosa, J.: 1980. Influencia de la temperatura ambiental y la humedad relativa sobre la tasa de concepción de vacas Holstein en condiciones cálido-húmedas Rev. Salud Anim. 2(3):129.

Restrepo Rivera Jairo.: 1995. Notas sobre agricultura orgánica y una crítica al modelo convencional. Agricultura Orgánica (1):8-14.

Rodríguez, E. (2000): Estudio de cinco especies forestales como postes vivos en sistemas de producción animal. Memorias IV Taller Internacional Silvipastoril. Los árboles y arbustos en la ganadería tropical. 20 nov, 2000. Estación Experimental de Pasto y Forrajes Indio Hatuey, Cuba.

Soca Mildrey, Simón L., Cáceres O. y Rivero L.: 1997. Variantes del uso del follaje de Leucaena leucocephala en un entorno agroecológico. III Encuentro Nacional de Agricultura Orgánica. Universidad Central L.V., Cuba.

Suárez J., Monzote Marta, Serrano D. y Fuentes Cheleny.: 1996. Integración agricultura-ganadería en un sistema agroecológico de una hectárea. II Simposio sobre agricultura sostenible. X Seminario Científico del INCA, La Habana.

Suárez J., Simón L. y Yepes I.: 1997. Uso de árboles y arbustos forrajeros en cercas vivas de La Habana y Matanzas. III Encuentro Nacional de Agricultura Orgánica, Universidad Central, L. V. Cuba.

Thatcher, W.:1974. Effect of season, climate, and temperature on reproduction and lactation. J. Dairy Sci. 57(3):360-368.

Urbina F., Eizaga F. y Dirinot F.:1996. La agricultura sustentable y su potencial en el trópico. II Simposio sobre agricultura sostenible. X Seminario Científico del INCA. La Habana.

Author's review

The author Luis Orlando Alba Gómez, PhD, Full Professor, Expert in Bovine Reproduction. Former Head of the Animal Reproduction Chair for 50 years at the Universidad Central de L.V. and José Martí in Sancti Spiritus, Cuba. He directed more than 30 Diploma Theses, 15 Specialization Theses and two PhDs in Veterinary Sciences. He has published 28 articles in journals and five scientific books.

a

b

www.ingramcontent.com/pod-product-compliance
Lightning Source LLC
Chambersburg PA
CBHW052259220526
45471CB00001B/407